I0405383

Ebola 2014

Leah E. Roberts

Published by Leah E. Roberts, MS at Smashwords

© Copyright 2014

This work is subject to Copyright.

No part of this publication may be reproduced, stored in a retrieval system or device or transmitted in any form or by any means, electronic, mechanical, photographic, or otherwise without the prior written permission of the author.

This eBook is licensed for your personal enjoyment only. This eBook may not be re-sold or given away to other people. If you would like to share this book with another person, please purchase an additional copy for each recipient. If you're reading this book and did not purchase it, or it was not purchased for your use only, then please return to your favorite eBook retailer and purchase your own copy. Thank you for respecting the hard work of this author.

Cover image by Leah E. Roberts using the following components:

Flight patterns By Jpatokal (Own work) [CC-BY-SA-3.0-2.5-2.0-1.0 (http://creativecommons.org/licenses/by-sa/3.0) or GFDL (http://www.gnu.org/copyleft/fdl.html)], via Wikimedia Commons

Precipitation map by USDA from http://www.pecad.fas.usda.gov/

and

"Ebola virus particles" by Thomas W. Geisbert, Boston University School of Medicine - PLoS Pathogens, November 2008 direct link to the image description page doi:10.1371/journal.ppat.1000225. Licensed under Creative Commons Attribution 2.5 via Wikimedia Commons - http://commons.wikimedia.org/wiki/File:Ebola_virus_particles.jpg#mediaviewer/File:Ebola_virus_particles.jpg

Contents

Introduction

Ebola has recently garnered the attention of the global community due to the magnitude and spread of the disease through countries in West Africa where it never had been seen. As the outbreak continued to spread, volunteer doctors and health workers from other countries became infected and were flown back to their home countries much to the protest of the citizens in their countries. Because of the lack of available and reputable knowledge for ordinary people outside of medicine, there has been a lot of fear, mistrust, and rumors that breed fear circulating. This outcome is not unlike that seen in Africa when the disease appeared in Guinea and then Liberia, followed by several other West African countries over the course of a year. This reference should provide both medical personnel needing a refresher on Ebola and everyone else who wishes to know facts a trustworthy resource that is free of unnecessary material.

Ebola belongs to the viral family known as Filoviridae, or filoviruses. Under this heading, there are 5 Ebola viruses, only one Marburg virus and a more newly discovered Lloviu virus. Many resources describe all of the other filoviruses at length so they will not be discussed here to avoid redundancy (Kuhn & Calisher, 2008; Olival & Hayman, 2014; WHO, 2014; CDC, 2014).

The significance of Ebola vs. other diseases is centered around the severity of the illness, the degree of profound human suffering involved with the disease process, the communicability, and the lack of proven treatments or prevention available and high mortality rates in victims. As of this writing, no approved drugs or vaccines are widely available. This ongoing outbreak that began in Guinea at the end of December, 2013 has gotten international attention. Media coverage has brought the potential for fear to every country on the planet via TV, newspapers, and of course, the internet. Many countries and even individual states have begun to develop protocol for dealing with Ebola on the chance that Ebola might reach their region via infected travelers. With open borders and often insufficient surveillance, it is easy to perceive how Ebola might enter a country via illegal immigrants and by air travel. There are not many places on Earth that cannot be accessed by airplanes in a fraction of an incubation period. The implications of a globally spread pandemic of this virus has many people who were never concerned about this virus grasping for knowledge as the statistics continue to rise (Atherstone, Roesel & Grace, 2014; Kuhn & Calisher, 2008).

Dr. Michael Katz of University of Washington has studied Ebola and genetic markers of the virus for over a decade and he says that none of the so-called 'known facts' about ebola can be certain because most of the studies referenced are based on the study of the virus in cell cultures and in animals (often virus adapted to the particular animal being used for the research like Guinea Pigs). Certain animal models have been shown to provide accurate outcomes when compared to observed human cases, but because we also see differences in the various aspects in humans such as onset of disease, severity and types of symptoms, and differences in genetic markers among others, there continues to be uncertainty even about our most solid beliefs pertaining to this virus (Graf, 2014). The best defense is for everyone to continually educate themselves about the disease and make educated decisions based on that knowledge and when opposing aspects occur, to readjust protocols where necessary.

Ebola Strains

As of this writing, there are five known species of Ebola viruses, of which four are known to cause illness in humans. These are Zaire (ZEBOV), Sudan (SEBOV, SUDV), Reston (REBOV), Bundibugyo (BEBOV, BDBV), and Tai Forest (TAEBOV). Tai forest virus was first referred to as Cote D' Ivoire, Ivory Coast (CIEBOV, ICEBOV). There is suggestion that the variant circulating in Guinea, Liberia, Sierra Leone, Nigeria, and Senegal, and possibly other countries is a new variant related to the ZEBOV, but as of this writing, it is being called ZEBOV (ScienceDaily, 2014). Ebola viruses are negative sense, enveloped RNA viruses. These characteristics are important for a number of scientific reasons, but also for methods of deactivating the virus and disinfection or decontamination. Hundreds of lineages of the strains are being discovered now which reveal the virus's ability to mutate and even recombine though it is not fully understood what the differences in the various lineages mean for virulence, infectivity, and other aspects important to the survival and ability to continue in cycles (Kuhn & Calisher, 2008; Public Health Agency of Canada, 2014; Gire et al., 2014).

Virus Stability

Ebola viruses can survive for several days in liquid or dried form especially in organic substances like blood, vomit, or feces (Leroy et al., 2004). They are stable at room temperature and can be preserved at 4°C for several days or even indefinitely at -70°C. The viruses can tolerate multiple freeze-thaw repetitions and still be successfully cultured in Vero cells (Kuhn & Calisher, 2008).

They are inactivated by heating at 60°C for 30-60 minutes (erring on the longer time for caution), boiling at rapid boil for 5 minutes, gamma irradiation (1.2 x 106 rads to 1.27 x 106 rads), or by ultraviolet-C radiation (Public Health Agency of Canada, 2014). The guidelines for cooking and boiling are open to interpretation and might be misconstrued; imagining this is referring to the virus alone undergoing these treatments, possibly on utensils, equipment or other non-edible supplies, and not necessarily the virus protected in muscle tissue (meat) being prepared for consumption. Heating is touched on again in the section on disinfection and decontamination. Pressure cooking with household pressure cookers has been utilized in early outbreaks successfully to sterilize instruments (AABB, 2009; Federation of American Scientists, 1998; Pattyn, 1978).

Additionally, Ebola viruses may be intentionally made more stable using the solution of stachyose, sucrose and polyetheleneimine (PEI) in prescribed amounts. Adding the viruses to this solution can allow the freezing and freeze-drying that preserves their infectivity and other characteristics. As a solution, the combination of substances act as a cryoprotectant which prevents damage from freezing, a lycoprotectant which prevents desiccation, and a thermoprotectant which protects the virus from thermal ranges +/- 40°C. Ultimately this activity would maintain virulence through freeze-drying which could be important for vaccine industry research, but is also dual-use in terms of creating a version of the virus that is more likely to remain suspended in air as a bioweapon which will be discussed in a later section about biological weapon concerns (Drew, 2012).

Transmission

The initial transmission to humans is historically environmental in nature either by eating, butchering or other contact with infected animals that allows the virus to contact mucosa, enter the bloodstream, or by ingestion. Transmission of Ebola viruses has traditionally been thought to be through close contact with blood and bodily fluids. Most references that have published transmission data have mimicked the same standards which have recently been changed on websites like the one for CDC for Ebola. Changes were hurriedly made on the public health agency webpages of many counties after the virus was imported into the US by a Liberian man which resulted in some unfortunate lessons about the disease and how patients should be screened and how care is managed among other aspects. Person to person transmission of EBOV involves contact with infected blood or bodily fluids. Unlike the transmission of HIV, all bodily fluids (blood, any component of blood, sweat, tears, mucous secretions, saliva, aqueous humor, breast milk, urine, feces, vomit, amniotic fluid, and semen) are infectious with EBOV. There are rumors of the virus penetrating intact skin, but as of this writing, there is no published data to support the theory of Ebola virus infecting intact skin. The suggestion might be that because the virus can replicate in hair follicles and can test positive periodically for antigen, that there might be some potential for transmission. One study in particular, following the outbreak in Kikwit, DRC noted the observation of copious numbers of Ebola viral particles found in human skin and lumina of sweat glands. That study attempted reproducing this phenomena in animal models unsuccessfully but noted that burial practices amplify this as an exposure and that infection of others from skin contact into skin lesions of naïve persons was observed. Spread of that volume of virus via hands that would then touch mucous membranes, micro-abrasions, wounds, or food is easy to acknowledge and viral counts of those who died of the disease would be extremely high. Available research suggests that the potential for transmission from intact infected skin to naïve intact skin is rare if not at all (Kuhn & Calisher, 2008).

In Africa, outbreaks have started after exposure to bush meat, butchering of bush meat, eating bush meat or exposure involving some contact with articles or foods contaminated by bats as noted above (UC Berkeley Events, 2014). After this index exposure, subsequent exposures occur with care and cleaning of those who are sick and showing symptoms, especially fever, and through ritual burial ceremonies. Patients find their way to medical facilities where the healthcare workers are not always expecting to see viral hemorrhagic fevers and upon first presumptions, these index patients are thought to have malaria, cholera, typhoid, yellow fever and even Lassa fever because they are accustomed to these cases, which begin with similar symptoms as Ebola except for the fever. Universal precautions in care are important even before a diagnosis because even if the patient does not have Ebola, they may potentially transfer a number of other often equally dangerous diseases to the caregivers. In health facilities, transmission has been amplified by the re-use of syringes, needles, and other medical supplies, absence of gloves, masks and other protection, and contact with the patients' skin and excretions and blood, especially before the virus is suspected. More recent observations suggest that either substandard training, incomplete knowledge of infection control, incorrect use of personal protective equipment (PPE) and removal of PPE have precipitated exposures in healthcare workers both in Africa and outside Africa (King, et al, 2014; Lagow, 2002; Howard, 2005; Stern, 2014).

Sexual transmission of Ebola has been documented and it is an important feature to be aware of for transmission. Later in the section about convalescents, there is more discussion on the persistence of virus in semen and vaginal secretions in convalescence, but it is worth additional emphasis that people are contracting the disease through sexual intercourse. If the virus is present in the bodily fluids it can be transmitted to a susceptible partner. Numerous reports have been published about both men and women transmitting the virus in convalesce to their partners but it is possible that they could be transmitting the disease before their symptoms are so extreme that they would not be interested in engaging in sexual intercourse. In order to determine just how soon sexual transmission can occur, it would be important to study the time required for virus to appear in semen and vaginal secretions in animal models that most closely resemble human models. Without this sort of information, it will be difficult to prove exactly when sexual contact is infectious, but it is wise to advise caution for sexual activity with anyone presenting early symptoms (Johnson, 2014; Rodriguez et al., 1999; Kuhn and Calisher, 2008; Howard, 2005).

There have been studies where reports of treatments by natural healers facilitated the spread of the virus to others and ultimately to themselves. Such a situation was the culprit in the spread of the virus in 2014 to Sierra Leone via the funeral of a traditional healer where at least 12 attendees to her funeral became sick. An earlier case was in 1995 where a man became ill following the hunting of chimpanzees where this species of NHP were found dead in paths and taken to eat, and butchered regardless. Many were infected from the butchering of the chimpanzees found dead, but one in particular had been a hunter by reports of his fellow villagers and sought treatment from a *Nganga*, which is a "natural healer" in DRC. This healer was treating via scarification where some instrument is used to make cuts in the skin which scar over and it is believed that in this process, the disease is released. After this, the Nganga, his assistant and patients that were subsequently treated by them were infected and 11 of 15 cases in the area died though it is not mentioned which patients or if they were the ones described as related by treatment to the Nganga (Pourrut et al., 2005). Numerous accounts of traditional healers falling ill have been reported during this 2014 outbreak as well.

There are clinical observations indicating a high rate of death in children of infected mothers whether that is due to breastfeeding, which is widely known to contain virus, or through other care methods, close contact, or by secondary incidences that arise from being orphaned by the death of the parents. Many references mention sharing a bed or room with an infected Ebola patient was the source of infection for a contact, which suggests an aerogenic transmission although no specific contact is mentioned in any of those references or in the current literature as of this writing. It is notable to also recall that many of the healthcare workers who treated patients in West Africa during this outbreak and fell ill themselves could not recall how or when they could have been exposed (Lupi & Tyring, 2003; Reuters, 2014; Stern, 2014).

The ability of Ebola and other filoviruses to be transmitted via airborne routes in natural environments and without adulteration is still heavily debated. Canadian investigator, Dr. Gary Kobinger, from the Special Pathogens Program, and his colleagues studied infection of ZEBOV in pigs in 2011 upon inspiration of reported transmission from pigs to Non-Human Primates (NHP) in a lab setting. Earlier reports from 2008 and also 2012 noted pigs being susceptible to EBOV infection. In their study, Kobinger and researchers exposed pigs to ZEBOV through their mucosa which resulted in high virus titers in the pigs' respiratory tracts and also virus shedding in the nasal mucosa of the pigs for up to 14 days after infection. This shows that aerosols created by the pigs through their snouts would contain virus and be an infection risk due to their ability to contaminate surfaces and in the short term – the air around them (Science Daily, 2011; Kobinger et al., 2011).

EBOV symptoms in pigs can be mistaken for other porcine respiratory illnesses just as EBOV disease symptoms in humans can look like Malaria and other diseases early on (Atherstone, Roesel & Grace, 2014). The importance of pigs and Ebola will be covered below in a dedicated section.

Studies done by Dr. Kobinger and his team in early 2014 in Canada remark about the rare occurrences where transmission through the air were observed and they resolve to a somewhat neutral position where they concluded, "Airborne transmission in natural outbreaks cannot be a common occurrence, and is possibly insignificant by the account of several reports". They then reference 5 studies which conclude to that effect. They followed by remarking that pigs were observed in their own prior research, infecting naïve NHPs via respiratory routes as they expelled the virus via coughing after which, they admit that, "Eventually, it will be important to assess the possibility of transmission between mucosally infected NHPs and naïve animals. In discussion, these researchers noted that pigs infected monkeys accidentally in the lab and assumed this was due to the close proximity of the cages which would allow droplets to make contact, but not so close to allow physical contact. They noted that in past experiments using the same species of NHPs (Macaques) and ZEBOV through injection which they presumed would replicate a 'natural infection' where virus entered the blood, they did not observe virus shedding through the mucosa of the NHPs, but in this accidental transmission, autopsies revealed virus in the lungs of the Macaques. No studies prove unequivocally that airborne transmission does not happen, and they do not deny it can happen; they only comment that it is not likely (Science Daily, 2011; Kobinger et al., 2011; Flohr, 2013).

The confusion around airborne transmission is in the interpretation. Most people relate to airborne transmission as being exposed to a pathogen through breathing. This is partially true, but scientists like to further define airborne in terms of the size of the inhaled particles. The reasoning is that particles of ideal airborne potential, according to USAMRIID (United States Army Research Institute for Infectious Diseases) being between 1 and 5 microns in diameter, will remain suspended in air longer and not settle to surfaces as fast as larger droplets. Additionally those smaller particles would be more capable of reaching the deep lungs where they would initiate infection. The size of droplets expelled by human test subjects in a study were found to be in the noted ideal range, 0.58-5.42 microns on average, with more than 82% falling between 0.74-2.12 microns (Yang et al., 2007). Aerosol transmissions can still occur with larger particles though, and even up to 100 micron particles can be inhaled, which in the case of Ebola could be significant with the contact to mucous membranes even if those particles do not reach deep into the trachea and lungs (Harriman & Brosseau, 2011). There has been a lot of discussion about the spread of Ebola through air in social media forums. There are still those who refuse to believe the virus can be spread through air and they have argued that they see no studies which prove that the virus replicates enough in the lung tissues that would allow easy exposures to occur via coughing, sneezing, and talking or breathing. Likewise, those who argue that Ebola can spread through the air describe cases where the transmission could reasonably have been via air and other cases where unexplained exposures occurred in those who had no known physical contact or exposures to infected bodily fluids. Until better studies have irrefutably concluded one way or the other, it is wise to be cautious and use adequate protection to avoid possible infection from this route.

The PDR Guide notes what they describe as 'potential aerogenic infection' where they describe a fatal inhalation as "400 plaque-forming units". In virology, PFUs refer to each viral particle that is capable of forming plaques, a beginning phase in infection; denoting that defective particles, if present are not counted. No description for dose necessary for infection in terms of plaque-forming units was noted but the Public Health Agency of Canada (as well as several other sources for infectious disease management and prevention) list an infectious dose as 1-10 viral organisms but with more virus in this loading dose, one would observe faster onset of symptoms due to more virus replicating exponentially (PDR Guide, 2002; Public Health Agency of Canada, 2014).

Current research being conducted in Monrovia by a team led by Dr. Peter Jahrling, Chief Scientist at the National Institutes of Allergy and Infectious Diseases, and a leading scientist for the research of Level 4 pathogens, is proving that the virus circulating in this outbreak has mutated in ways that allow the virus to replicate faster and to greater numbers than before (Belluz, 2014). This trend may not be long lived; however, as evidence from genomic structures called "replikins" shows a downward trend. Replikins are amino acid sequences observed in all pathogens that can be studied from sequenced genomes of the various pathogens. Researchers at Replikins Ltd. observed incremental increases in the replikins of sequenced Ebola viruses in the period from 1995 through 2012, but a sixteen-fold increase was seen in 2013. Work with replikins relating to Influenza viruses revealed these kinds of rises prior to all of the major historical Flu outbreaks, and suggest that the huge increase in replikins seen with Ebola was predictive of the 2013-2014 outbreak. Continued observation of these sequences throughout the outbreak in 2014 has shown a significant drop which researchers are claiming equates to a trend for slower replication than has been reported thus far (Bogoch & Bogoch, 2011; Borsanyi, 2014; Drug Discovery and Development Magazine, 2014).

Cultural Importance

The socio-cultural aspects of each region that is affected by the Ebola outbreak impact the potential progression of the disease or its control. There are more cultural components that have the ability to amplify disease transmission than simply burial practices. Throughout Africa, the preparation of a body for burial is a ritual in and of itself. Most often tasked to the women in families, the preparation may involve washing the body and sometimes body cavities depending on the specific culture. This washing by family members is not only a practice of African people; it is done in Islamic cultures throughout Africa and also globally, but it is also practiced in variation by indigenous tribes and even Jewish cultures (Haglage, 2014).

When considering a body that has died from Ebola, depending on the condition of the skin, severity of disease, and conditions that led to death there are considerations that should be brought to light. If the patient died with patches of desquamated skin and hemorrhages or fluid seeping through, washing the body could be a very high-risk task, especially when spraying or splashing may create aerosols. Any residues of blood from the nose, mouth, ears and genital openings will be infectious as well as any residues remaining on the skin from feces or vomit.

In addition to washing, the body may be rubbed with various oils or herbs thought to infer some power or blessing to the dead and then the body is dressed in special clothes. Funerals can last several days depending on the status of the deceased person and have large groups of people attending who touch the body, touch and kiss the face of the body, and pray over it among other things. In some areas, relatives and friends of the deceased will pretend as the person is still alive in aspects such as sharing a cigarette with them or other ritualistic acts. In some cases, family members of the dead will cut the hair and trim the finger nails and toe nails of the deceased as part of the preparation for burial (Borio et al, 2002). Hand washing bowls are shared among the guests and can provide additional means for spreading the disease (Haglage, 2014; Hewlett & Hewlett, 2008; IRIN News, 2014).

Other more dangerous rituals involve the widow of dead men drinking the water that is used to wash her husband's dead body. The family of the dead man supposedly expects the widow to participate in this ritual to prove her innocence in his cause of death so if she refuses, she is suspected for murdering her husband and will have to move away with any children she has to prevent their own murders (Canada: Immigration and Refugee Board of Canada, 2012).

To avoid this unnecessary exposure, it is important for community leaders and tribal elders as well as any others with trusted positions in the community to gather with the people of the community and educate them about these and other risks. Any burial practices that result in exposure to blood or other body fluids must be halted or changed in some way to avoid the exposures. It could be possible to alter rituals to make them acceptable for infection control while still preserving the dignity and respect of the deceased and their family. A good example of this interaction is given by MSF in their article about a Liberian nurse, Eric, who died from Ebola. His funeral was a very large gathering where the man's brother and the priest along with an MSF health promoter all gathered to explain Ebola and why people get infected, what people can do to avoid infection, why it is so dangerous to touch the body and then they pleaded with the people to ignore the rumors, to get treatment if they feel sick, to report deaths and to learn from and cooperate with the health workers. This sort of community solidarity is needed to bolster trust and sense of community which will help to stop the continuation of infection chains (MSF, 2014).

A study that analyzed an Ebola outbreak in Masindi, Uganda in 2000 traced the index patient of a secondary outbreak involved in spread of the disease to other towns and it noted where the index patient and her family were stigmatized even after they had lived in their village for at least ten years with those same neighbors. The index patient and her family had moved there from Kenya years before, but when the disease began spreading amongst them and not immediately to the neighbors, the family felt they were being poisoned by the neighbors and lived clustered together in one home to avoid contact with neighbors. It was not until the eldest son of the index patient died that they listened to the driver of a community surveillance vehicle who held up a newspaper noting that many others were sick and dying of this disease and it was not the result of poisoning. The community was involved here to provide food and allow the family to get their water close to their homes to prevent spreading the disease to others in markets (Borchert et al., 2011).

The inclusion of community leaders is of paramount importance because simply explaining this to the people may not get them to understand the concepts enough to change their routines and behaviors. Having cultural modification starting with elders and leaders will fill gaps where lack of literacy in populations had been a barrier (Hewlett & Hewlett, 2008; MSF, 2014).

Many regions of Africa have similar beliefs about their burial rituals which agree that if no ritual is done or if it is not done properly, then the soul of the dead will remain unhappy or not cross over to non-physical or afterlife, and so, will haunt the family, bring them bad fortune, or bestow similar fate upon them (Hewlett & Hewlett, 2008). Finding respectful alternative methods to use in burial rituals could make the process including needed infection control measures somewhat more acceptable. The addition of 0.05% bleach to the hand washing water, providing gloves and other protective equipment and community training on avoiding exposures when tending to the dead for family members who insist on continuing burial rituals could be helpful.

Other cultural routines and social norms should be changed too, such as hand-shaking, hugging when greeting others, kissing on cheeks, and other contact-based greetings. Something like smiling with a nod or a bow as is done in some Asian cultures would still convey respect while preserving the need to avoid contact with others. This alteration of greetings would have the added benefit of keeping distance between people and act as a barrier of sorts in the event of potential 'aerogenic' transmissions (covered in the previous section). With a disease like Ebola, the possibility of transmission by any means should hold attention and not be ignored (Brosseau & Jones, 2014).

Long-held beliefs that have been handed down through many generations are not easily or abruptly changed without help from the entire community. In America, we used to believe that smoking cigarettes was not harmful but now, due to decades of research and the debilitation, suffering of smoking-related disease, and death of many thousands, beliefs about cigarettes have changed but there are still many thousands of people who continue to smoke even knowing it may one day kill them. Rituals, like social norms are passed to children for generations and are largely born from observations (seeing is believing); so if the observation is one where people enter the local hospital and either do not come out or they come out in a body bag, then the thoughts and relative beliefs provoked about hospitals can be that avoiding the hospitals can prevent death. That kind of belief is partially responsible for why this 2014 outbreak was allowed to get so bad before health workers could manage it. Control of Ebola outbreaks largely relies on epidemiology and contact tracing which requires trust from the people in the communities and participation of community leaders and elders (IRIN News, 2014; Mark, 2014).

Where the outbreak goes that people know about the implications of the disease and transmission, fear still sets in and the people may rush into hospitals when they develop minor symptoms because they are worried they may have Ebola. The observation of 'worried well' has been appreciated in other epidemics and even in the US. A perfect example of this is when the Anthrax letters were mailed and many people thought they could be exposed just because they received mail or because they lived in a town where others reported being infected or exposed. The burden of the worried well can easily overwhelm healthcare facilities. Thinking of Ebola being silently brought into the US, Europe, Australia, and other industrialized countries and considering the worried well, there would not even need to be a real exposure to see how that would play out. Someone with intent to create worry or even terror in a population (truly a terrorist) could set up a believable scenario to include a release of Ebola in an airplane, at a sporting event, or a crowded mall on a busy shopping day and the fear would drive the worried well to seek treatment. This would be a victory for the terrorist and no exposure would have even occurred (Collingwood, 2007; Stone, 2007).

Symptoms

Symptoms reported by Zairian doctor Ngoi Mushola from the 1976 outbreak were: fever with frequent vomiting of black blood, (denoting the partially digested blood that may have begun to seep into the stomachs of victims to be somewhat digested before nausea overcame them), bloody stools and nose bleeds. The initial patients who presented with these signs were thought to have Yellow Fever; that is until their certificates proved vaccine-induced immunity for Yellow Fever (Howard, 2005). It is these kinds of documented cases of Ebola that demand urgent attention from the global community. A well-documented case of a Russian lab scientist who was infected after pricking her palm with a contaminated needle reveals just how frightening the disease can be. Her condition appeared positive for the first six days, but from day 7 on, her condition deteriorated despite treatment with hyperimmune equine serum and good supportive care. She died with multiple organ failure while still conscious. She was described as being apathetic and weak near her time of death, but because she was still conscious, her case indicates the unmentionable human suffering that occurs with this disease (Kuhn & Callisher, 2008).

Symptoms of the disease vary depending on the initial health of the victim, other concurrent diseases or health issues, immune-competence, loading viral dose, route of transmission and possibly other aspects. Following an incubation period of between 2 and 21 days, symptoms begin. What is most often observed is 4-16 days of incubation with a mean of 7 days. It has been reported in several documents that infection by injection or other means to deliver the virus directly into blood shortens the incubation time between 2-6 days. Infections that involve other exposures like via the mouth, mucous membranes or other close contact tend to cause symptoms in a longer period averaging about 9 days. And experimental exposures using exponentially greater loading doses than the LD-50 (amount required to ensure half of the exposed will die) symptoms can be seen in just hours in lab animals (Ryabchikova & Price, 2004; Atherstone, Roesel & Grace, 2014).

Symptoms that have been observed in previous outbreaks vary according to time passed since the initial exposure, speed and efficiency of virus replication, loading dose, immune status of the host, and general health of the host among other aspects. The infectious dose for filoviruses including Ebola is considered to be one virus particle. Likewise, the LD-50 is also one virus particle. One filovirus particle is capable of infecting the first cell in a susceptible host that begins the infection that often ends in death (Ryabchikova & Price, 2004).

There has been debate about the incubation period, which is described as being between 2 and 21 days. It can be explained, although sounding vague, that 95% of confirmed Ebola cases develop symptoms between day 1 and day 21, but 98% of confirmed Ebola cases (including the 95% just noted) may have incubation periods between 1 and 42 days. This makes the actual number of days confusing to many people who have discussed this in social media groups and has raised concerns about the safety regarding shorter vs. longer isolation of suspected cases. The guidelines adopted are based on the research which notes most cases are apparent with symptoms in 21 days or less and the costs the benefits vs cost of isolating suspected cases past 21 days has been agreed upon as being inadequate. WHO guidelines require 2 tests for Ebola, 48 hours apart to test negative in order to classify an infected patient as a cured or convalescent, and Ebola-negative (Jayalakshmi, 2014; Kuhn & Calisher, 2008).

Initially – weakness, frontal headache – spreading to the back of the head (often crushing headache), radiating muscle aches, joint pain that begins in the large joints, dehydration, hiccups, sensitivity to light, vertigo, fever, and sore throat; these symptoms are followed by vomiting, diarrhea, abdominal pain, conjunctival injection (reddening of the white of the eyes), rashes and bleeding. Abdominal pain precedes the diarrhea which is often around 5 days following the onset of symptoms. Abdominal pain is often severe with palpation, but if palpation can be tolerated, it reveals an enlarged liver. There was a standing notation among public health agencies that the fever should be at least 101.5 to avoid isolation of someone who is not infected with Ebola, which may pose other problems but may prevent unnecessary scrutiny and testing. Newer guidelines based on observations in the US cases involving nurses infected while caring for the US index patient repeal the notion that a fever must be present in order to suspect

Ebola virus disease. It is possible that the earlier guidelines were based on the premise that PCR would most often not detect Ebola until there was a titer high enough to cause the fever, which occurs after a cascade of cellular reactions involving the immune system cells. Chest pains are also seen with Ebola virus disease where they are not with Marburg virus disease (PBS, 2014; UC Berkeley Events, 2014; Kuhn & Calisher, 2008; PDR Guide, 2002). Because symptoms such as fatigue might be passed off as unimportant before more severe symptoms are present, the disease could be given more opportunities to spread before it is acknowledged. This could help to explain some exposures where people cannot recall exposure to others. There is debate about transmission via those with sub-clinical infections which will be covered later in this text.

Hiccups are an odd symptom that was noted in about 15% of the confirmed cases during the Kikwit, DRC outbreak that indicated a fatal outcome. Hiccups were also observed in epidemic proportions during the 1918 Influenza pandemic and are now considered one of the most important symptoms in recognizing Ebola virus disease outbreaks. As noted later in this text, the presence of hiccups as a symptom of the-then-undiagnosed illness in this outbreak was what triggered the response for Ebola (Jayalakshmi, 2014; Kuhn & Calisher, 2008; Stern, 2014).

Later symptoms seen about 5-7 days after first signs have been – conjunctival hemorrhage and jaundice, pharyngitis, bleeding gums, mouth and lip ulcers, bleeding of intestinal tract and esophageal tract resulting in the vomiting of blood and diarrhea containing blood, non-menstrual vaginal bleeding, miscarriage of pregnancies with unusually copious bleeding, hypotension from loss of blood volume, renal failure and the late-stage symptoms in those who rarely survive include a normalizing of temperature, followed by multiple-organ failure and shock. Myoclonia, which is involuntary, non-rhythmic contractions in facial muscles have been observed and also the development of a mask-like face with deep-set eyes near the end stages of the disease. Additionally, stupor and a state of confusion is seen. The rashes begin as pinpoint dark red papules around the base of hairs on the face, torso and inside of arms. In a day or so, these rashes spread and are termed *maculopapular*, where there are both flat reddened areas and slightly raised red areas making up the rash, which can become confluent. Sometimes the rashes on the skin become hemorrhages in between the layers of skin that eventually desquamate, or separate the layers of skin creating large blood-blister like patches on the skin (PBS, 2014; UC Berkeley Events, 2014; Kuhn & Calisher, 2008; PDR Guide, 2002).

Pregnant women frequently abort their pregnancy and it is of note that pregnant women in general, with an altered immune system may be more susceptible to fatal infections with Ebola and other filoviruses. This phenomenon is shared with Lassa fever and accounts for the possible misdiagnosis for Lassa in West Africa where Lassa is expected (Kuhn & Calisher, 2008; Gire et al, 2012). Data about EVD in pregnant women has been scantily reported. During this outbreak, 2 women who presented with EVD during pregnancy were treated at the Médecins Sans Frontières (MSF) Ebola treatment centre in Guéckedou, Guinea. The age and circumstances of both women were quite different but their outcomes were similar in that they both recovered and they both had still-born babies and very high viral counts in the amniotic fluid. The first woman had responded to her treatment and was free of symptoms in just 6 days, tested negative for 2 Ebola tests around day 10 but on day 11 spiked a high fever and reported absence of fetal movement. An amniocentesis revealed the high viral count in the fluid. She was induced into labor and vaginally delivered a still-born baby. The baby also tested positive for EVD in both cases. The second woman was much younger but due to scarring of her genital region that resulted from severe female genital mutilation, her treatment was complicated and had to be improvised (Baggi et al., 2014).

On the cellular level, macrophages, which are directly involved with the blood system and immunity, are the primary target of filoviruses, although they are capable of infecting many other kinds of cells as well such as hepatocytes, adrenal cortical cells, endothelial cells and fibroblasts. When the Ebola virus attaches to a cell, it has the capability to shield its identity via mechanisms in the GP gene (a region called the 'mucin region') at the point of attachment on the cell that make it invisible to the MHC (major histocompatibility complex). The MHC cells are the ones that flag down killer T-cells which would be the first T-cells to mount an offense, but since there is no signal with the shielding of the filovirus, no response is summoned and this leads to the evasion of both humoral and cellular immune responses as the virus is left to replicate quietly (Francia, 2010; Sompayrac, 2008). There are additional roles where the GP gene helps viral entry into host cells. In experiments using either human or porcine blood vessels that are held in a medium, this glycoprotein exhibited massive endothelial cell loss in 48 hours post infection and an increase of vascular permeability. The GP gene of the virus is therefore likely contributory to the hemorrhage seen in late stage Ebola virus disease. There are two forms of GP protein synthesized by the GP gene, one is a surface protein that aids in the entry into cells, and the other has cytotoxic effects (Yang et al, 2000). There is also the VP 35 which is a Type I interferon antagonist and the VP30, and L gene, both of which are part of a replicase complex (Leroy et al, 2002). These cells release a cascade of mediators like interleukins, gamma-interferon, and tumor necrosis factor (TNF) and other substances related to inflammation that impair lung microcirculation, impair immunity, affect blood clotting, blood vessel permeability and more. Observations made of experimental animals revealed accumulation of neutrophils, which cause alveolar thrombosis, in the lungs where extensive damage to tissues occurred. Neutrophils can trigger Acute Respiratory Distress Syndrome (ARDS) in other diseases. Filoviral diseases are associated with intravascular inflammation in humans and animals where the immune system is somehow functionally compromised. The processes of disease happen in much the same way in all bodily organs (Ryabchikova & Price, 2004; Howard, 2005).

Doctors working during the 1995 outbreak in Kikwit, Zaire, (now DRC) commented about the disabling mental status of patients during later stages of disease. Many who suffered severe hemorrhagic disease and recovered have little recollection about the end stages. Health workers and others observing patients in those late stages described the patient as having a sort of dementia which indicates cerebral involvement (Kuhn & Calisher, 2008; Howard, 2005). In the current outbreak, a doctor who tested positive for EVD in Sierra Leone was flown back to the US and treated at the Emory University Hospital where his condition deteriorated to the point of kidney and other organ failure. He was put on dialysis and a ventilator which was able to keep him alive while his body utilized convalescent serum donated by another survivor of the disease. During his experience, he noted encephalitic symptoms and relative loss of memory in the time he spent in the facility in dire illness but he fortunately recovered (Grady, 2014). Additional psychiatric sequelae have included confusion, anxiety, restless and aggressive behavior. This is important to caregivers who may observe strange behavior or even combative behavior as can be observed in patients with senile dementia. With impaired mental status, patients may forget where they are, why they are there, and become difficult to care for or manage; worse, may become a threat to health care workers and others as combative patients may breech the PPE garments that workers wear for protection.

Collectively, those patients who experience a second spike in fever around 38 °C and 100.4°F, which would occur around days 12-14 of the illness and can precede multiple organ failure, often die. Those who survive through day 16 of the illness usually recover (Kuhn & Calisher, 2008; Howard, 2005; PDR Guide, 2002).

Lab results testing a variety of markers in blood reveal the following in Ebola disease: EHR, Erythrocytes and Leukocytes climb in number as disease progresses while Lymphocyte numbers plummet.Thrombocytopenis is observed and there is a drop in hemoglobin, protein and albumin. Creatine, bilirubin, SGOT & SGPT all rise. Fibrinogin is normal on the first day, but clots no longer form after day 13 in those who eventually succumb (Kuhn & Callisher, 2008).

Diagnosis

Diagnosis is based on a positive result from an Ebola virus-specific test or immunoglobulin-specific test, and can be delayed when the disease outbreaks begin especially when there is a lack of suspicion of the virus as the cause of illnesses. Depending on how much time has passed since the exposure, the kind of exposure and viral load among other possible aspects, the kind of test used may be different. PCR (Polymerase Chain Reaction) tests may not reveal a positive result on a positive patient until at least three days following onset of symptoms (AABB, 2014). Viral mRNA, however, can be detected in blood samples as early as 7 hours after infection. RT-PCR (Reverse Transcriptase Polymerase Chain Reaction) can be performed fast and used to find viral RNA with high specificity (Howard, 2005).

Immunoglobulins tested for are usually IgG and IgM. The IgG are the smallest of the five types of antibodies and also the most abundant. IgG antibodies can be found in any bodily fluid. IgG is the only kind of antibody that can cross the placenta in pregnancy. IgGs are produced several days after the immune system identifies an infection and mounts a response with IgMs and other immune system cells. Presence of IgG in body fluids often signifies the pathogens causing the infection are mostly gone. IgM antibodies are the largest kind of antibody; they are the first to appear as a result of infection when the infection is occurring for the first time in the host and can be found in blood or lymph fluid. IgM antibodies act to also encourage other cells of the immune system to secrete substances that fend off pathogens and the majority are produced in the spleen (Coico & Sunshine, 2009).

In some accounts of Ebola patients that were documented from the Kikwit, Zaire outbreak in 1995, IGM lasted for at least 168 days after the onset of illness. IgG was present between 6 and 18 days after the onset of illness and they were still detected in blood samples as long as 749 days. Viral antigen was no longer observed after 7-16 days in blood (Kuhn & Calisher, 2008).

In the areas of Africa where the virus has traditionally surfaced, other diseases with similar early symptoms are more common. Diseases like Cholera, Typhoid, Yellow Fever, Malaria, and in West Africa, Lassa Hemorrhagic Fever all begin with the same flu-like symptoms. Often, when the Ebola virus is suspected, patients are considered "suspected cases" until laboratory tests can be sent out and confirm presence of the virus. Early in the disease, blood can be drawn and sent to competent labs for the following tests: Antigen-capture enzyme-linked immunosorbent assay (ELISA) testing, IgM ELISA, PCR, and Virus isolation. Virus isolation is best done with blood or liver specimens. ELISA tests are useful in the acute phase of illness to detect viral antigen substances which would not necessarily be present early on. Filoviruses do not agglutinate the erythrocyte cells in humans (or guinea pigs) so IFA and antigen-capture ELISA would be a preferred and safe test for diagnosing Ebola until a rapid field-compatible test can be approved for use. Organs like spleen, liver, and kidneys often are found with the highest concentrations of virus (Kuhn & Calisher, 2008). Late-stage disease or after recovery, labs can test blood samples for IgM and IgG antibodies. For deceased patients, Immunohistochemistry testing, PCR, and virus isolation can be used. Many other tests exist for detection of Ebola, but there is optimism for approval of those tests that provide rapid or even instant results which will improve control of spread as well as the care and likely recovery of the patients (Kuhn & Calisher, 2008; CDC, 2014). It would be pertinent to test the deceased for virus isolation from those body fluids (such as semen) known to still contain virus in convalescence as it would make sense that the virus would remain there at least 48 hours after death considering the time bodies are considered to be infective. Also because the spleen tends to have high virus replication, this organ would be useful in finding virus if other tests fail and there is strong suspicion of Ebola diagnosis and other methods of testing give negative results.

False negative tests have occurred enough times during this outbreak to command the need for at least 2 tests for confirmation both to diagnose the disease and to declare a patient free of the disease. Many instances have been reported and discussed in the social media channels like LinkedIn, Facebook, and Twitter citing articles and reports of patients being sick with obvious symptoms and being given a negative test result using PCR tests. One particular report noted a man becoming sick after a trip to Kenema, Sierra Leone but when he was taken by ambulance to an Ebola treatment center his test came back negative and he was returned to his village. His condition worsened as his family and others tried to care for him and treat him with traditional means which involved herbs as they thought he was sick because of witchcraft. At least 30 others were infected as a result of this false negative test (McCordic, 2014).

There are several companies working to develop faster tests which could be used in the field, so to speak, which do not involve sending samples to labs far away and rather offer more instant gratification and faster diagnosis; therefore, faster treatment for patients. One company in particular, Shenzhen Puruikang Biotech Company in Shenzhen, Guangdong Province of China has produced a test kit which is able to detect any Ebola virus in a sample within 3-4 hours, compared to several days to a week or more for shipping samples to labs. Their tests use a chemical solution that reacts with specific nucleic acids in Ebola viruses and causes the color of the solution to change. The company said back in August, that they got the green light to mass produce these tests for use in Africa's ongoing outbreak. As of this writing, there have been no reports of successes or failures in English language media. However, a company in Colorado, USA, named Corgenix has worked with researchers at Tulane University to develop a rapid test taking about 15 minutes for results and it contains the patient sample so there is less exposure risk to healthcare workers (Zhin, 2014; Chen, 2014).

A French company, Vedalab, has developed a testing device that is designed to work much like home pregnancy tests which would provide a quick and accurate test result in the field without the need for any additional equipment. Their test, called "eZYSCREEN" can test blood, plasma, or urine and provide a result in just 15 minutes (Wasserman, 2014). There is hope that it can be put to good use to help rapidly diagnose and allow treatment of those who need it most in Africa, but it is reasonable to assume this test could be used to screen those passengers arriving in new countries from an affected area when there is suspicion of Ebola Virus Disease.

A newer rRT-PCR test recently received FDA authorization for emergency use but it still requires a specialized machine to process the samples and give results. This test says it can provide results in just over 3 hours (PRNewswire, 2014).

Numerous other tests are being developed that claim to have results in as few as fifteen minutes. At least three of those testing companies hope to have marketable products available within 2-3 years, possibly in time to meet needs of subsequent outbreaks.

Treatment

Until this outbreak, treatment has been limited to general supportive care such as replacing coagulation factors in the blood, administering heparin if disseminated intravascular coagulation (DIC) is present (which is debatable by some), attention to intravascular volume (to prevent shock which can be responsible for fatal cases), electrolytes, nutrition, and comfort. It has been the observation in thousands of cases, that supportive care done well can make a difference in the patient's survival. Pharmacological interventions may include Nucleoside Analog Inhibitors of SAH, various hyper-immune globulins and equine-derived IgG which was found to prolong life, but not so much as to prevent death. There are many new and cutting-edge medicines, treatment regimens, and vaccines in development as a result of the urgency created by this outbreak. Scientists are also examining older medicines for potential benefit to Ebola patients. Selective estrogen receptor modulators (SERMs) are one such class of drug being studied for its strong inhibitive effects on Ebola virus infections (Johansen et al., 2013). Convalescent plasma was used during the outbreak in Kikwit, DRC (formerly Zaire) in 1995 using whole blood transfusions on 8 patients and only one of those patients died. Convalescent serum or plasma use was still controversial in the first six months or more into this outbreak, but it seems that attitudes have changed as we observe convalescent serum being used in every case possible and also the serum is being saved in sort of banks in the US. Techniques are also being developed that ensure other pathogens are filtered out. Additionally, medicines that help to provide comfort such as anti-nausea and pain medications are helpful (King et al., 2014; PBS, 2014; VICE News, 2014).

Favoring adequate and optimal supportive care, newer case reports involving patients with Ebola who had been evacuated to developed countries for care show how routine supportive care was successful even in severe cases of Ebola where encephalopathy, respiratory failure and gram-negative septicemia was present. That supportive care included ICU treatment, a ventilator, broad spectrum antimicrobial therapy and high-volume fluid resuscitation. In one particular case report, the patient was in grave condition entering ICU care but survived with that care even though virus was still present in his urine at day 30, in his sweat at day 40 which were detected using PCR. Cultures of his plasma had virus up to 14 days (Kreuls, et al, 2014).

On the heels of using convalescent serum, there are about 50 genetically modified cows being studied in South Dakota that were engineered to produce human antibodies. These kinds of cattle were studied recently for their ability to produce antibodies to hantavirus which has been known to kill human hosts in many regions of the world. The herd has been vaccinated against Ebola, according to a recent article with NBC News, and tests thus far have revealed high quantities of human-antibodies to Ebola. The group, working with USAMRIID (US Army Research Institute for Infectious Diseases) hopes this antibody can be harvested and used to treat Ebola victims at a rate close to 500 to 1,000 human doses per month per animal (Fox, 2015).

Dr. Gobee Logan in rural Liberia used the HIV drug Lamivudine to treat his Ebola patients which resulted in startling positive improvements in 12 of 14 patients who received it. Those 12 people were able to start taking that drug within the first 5 days of their onset of illness whereas the two who died took it between days 5 & 8 denoting an urgency for a window in the progression of illness for this to work. Lamivudine is a nucleoside analog drug that helps prevent the replication of virus, but also carries various side effects. This drug is used in treatment of HIV, Hepatitis B and other viral illnesses but it is noted that over the course of several years of use, there is tendency for resistance to occur (Cohen, 2014; LiverTox, 2014). It would be interesting to learn about those in Africa who had been taking this drug as well as other anti-viral medications to treat HIV, their exposure to Ebola-infected patients, incidence of Ebola infections in those taking anti-viral medication prior to infection, and possible prevention of the disease in those on anti-viral medications.

Focusing on the cellular level pathology of Ebola Virus Disease (EVD) researchers explain that the endothelial injury resulting from cascades of immune reactions, release of toxic substances within the tissue, and inflammatory responses that all culminate to the development of disseminated intravascular coagulation (DIC), and end-stage multiple-organ hemorrhage are similar to those seen in sepsis. Using melatonin for treatment could potentially help protect EVD patients because it is known to be a potent anti-inflammatory agent, free-radical scavenger that has been proven effective for protecting those cells targeted by EBOV which are endothelial cells, which are located all over the body. Additionally, melatonin exhibits many other protective effects relating to coagulation. They theorize that administering melatonin in doses of 20mg or more several times a day could therefore prevent these cascades from resulting in the fatal damage seen in EVD fatalities. Melatonin has a very high safety rating and has successfully treated even newborns with sepsis (Tan, Reiter & Manchester, 2014).

A newer drug ZMAPP was used experimentally in the cases of two US doctors who fell ill while working in Ebola clinics in West Africa. The drug uses three man-made antibodies to the Ebola virus which are grown in genetically-modified tobacco plants. The drug was claiming 100% protection for NHPs but so far, three who got the drug lived while two others who also received the drug died (Boseley, 2014).

In December, 2014, a drug called FX06, initially created for treatment of "vascular leak syndrome" by a company in Austria was successfully used to treat a 38 year old male doctor who was infected with Ebola while treating patients in Sierra Leone. The patient had severe multiple organ failure when first admitted to a German facility at 5 days past his onset of symptoms, but after just 3 days of the treatment combined with supportive care, broad-spectrum anti-microbial therapy and renal replacement therapy, the patient recovered (Wolf, et al., 2014).

When considering drug therapies, it is important to consider the dosages and differences in metabolism for children and the elderly as opposed to those for young and middle-aged adults.

Transfusions are also recommended for cases with severe bleeding. IV fluids can be given for hypotension in large amounts to prevent shock. If other measures are not showing response in the patient, dopamine can be administered, followed by norepinephrine if no response to the dopamine (PDR Guide, 2002).

Four lab workers in Russia with exposures to EVOB (one with a high-risk exposure) were treated with a combination of goat-derived anti-Ebola immunoglobulin and recombinant interferon-alfa-2 and all four of them recovered (King et al., 2014).

In 2014, biofiltration of human blood was done with an experimental "Hemipurifier" device made by Aethlon Medical. The device was designed to filter out viruses and immunosuppressive proteins from the blood of a patient who was sick with Ebola. This device was proven useful in patients with HIV and HCV (Hepatitis C Virus) in India and recently helped a patient in Sierra Leone who was a Ugandan doctor that became infected and progressed to multiple organ failure to recover (Helio Infectious Disease News, 2014).

Numerous studies focusing on vaccines and therapeutic pharmaceuticals are being conducted presently worldwide and now with even more urgency as this 2014 outbreak continues to gain momentum. Vaccine development is not covered here, but it is worthy to note the common observation in outbreaks as well as in lab experiments using animals that sometimes, prior infection does not confer immunity, rather, a phenomena dubbed "early death phenomenon" is seen where certain antibodies were thought to enhance virus-entry into the host cells (Kuhn & Calisher, 2008; Ryabchikova, 2004).

There are now a number of articles that suggest a period of immunity to Ebola following the survival of an infection with Ebola, but studies that definitively prove the immunity is protective against a future infection upon challenge with the same strain or another strain have not been published as of this writing. Attention to this theory of protective immunity should be further explored before assuming it to be true based on observations of other disease models.

It is likely that in a future revision there may be inclusion of any vaccines developed that become approved and deemed to be safe and effective if such a vaccine is made available.

Recovery

Events that happen in the immune system of the patient during the early response to the infection determine whether the patient will recover or die from this disease. Recovery relies on precise humoral and cellular immune responses which can be observed by the early presence of IgM and IgG followed by activation of cytotoxic cells. In those patients who die from the disease, humoral immune responses are impaired early among other characteristics that are followed by cell death in all of the organ systems (Leroy et al., 2000; Lupi & Tyring, 2003).

Certain genetic markers (alleles that correspond to immune cells called CD8+ lymphocytes) have been shown in lab experiments, to be indicative of reliable predictions of survival or death from Ebola. People in Uganda, during the 2000-2001 outbreak of SEBOV, who had any of these alleles (B67, B13, or B42) were more likely to die from an infection of Ebola whereas those who had these (B35, B7, B14, and B40) were much more likely to live. In the area of extremes, all of those with the B67 allele died from their infection. In the selection of participants with SEBOV disease, two had a combination of one "good" allele and one "bad" allele, but the disease outcome for those patients was not revealed. These markers could have potential to predict a fatal or non-fatal outcome in patients as they are admitted to a treatment center and therefore aid in tailoring more appropriate care (Sanchez, Wagoner & Rollin, 2007). It may be possible to adjust care for those carrying the alleles for a bad outcome in ways that could change their genetically-predicted fate especially concerning the use of newly developed drugs such as ZMAPP used experimentally for two American doctors who were infected in the middle of the year, 2014.

As patients recover, they need nutrition and supportive care to continue with attention to hydration. Patients recovering may continue to develop inflammatory diseases such as Uveitis, orchitis, pericarditis, joint pain, and experience deafness and psychosis. Arthralgia of the large joints lasted as long as 21 months in cases documented in the Kikwit, Zaire outbreak and the antibody levels were higher in patients who complained of joint pain. Additionally, convalescent patients may continue to suffer from recurrent hepatitis and psychosis requiring continuation of varying care. They also suffer from extreme fatigue which may impose problems for returning to a job. Headaches and hair loss are also reported (Kuhn & Calisher, 2008; Atherstone, Roesel & Grace, 2014). Newer reports concerning survivors in this outbreak are detailing reproductive issues such as amenorrhea (where menstruation ceases for some period of time) and erectile dysfunction with possible impotency (IRIN News, 2014).

Many convalescents may develop severe depression and need psychological care because in parts of Africa, cultural beliefs and stigma reign over medical knowledge of disease enjoyed by more industrialized countries and patients report going home to a pile of ashes where neighbors burned down their homes and all of their possessions in fear of somehow spreading the sickness. Ebola disease is also stigmatized because many cultures believe sickness is caused by witchcraft or that sickness happens to bad people; meaning they must have committed an awful crime of humanity to be cursed with such an illness so others do not want to associate with a survivor fearing they too may be cursed (Hewlett & Hewlett, 2008; Kuhn & Calisher, 2008; Hewlett & Hewlett, 2008; Lupi & Tyring, 2003).

With the rising numbers of survivors of Ebola, it could be a logical solution for those survivors who are being avoided by their home communities to come together and build their own communities. Here survivors could care for one another without stigma and adopt surviving children which could also give new hope and life to those children who were orphaned by the disease. A community of survivors might also be helpful in their local clinics as well as in the care of orphaned children, provided they have immunity following their convalescence.

Patients who are recovering are still infectious through their body fluids particularly semen and breast milk among other body fluids and should have exit-counseling to help them understand the importance of avoiding contact which could infect others even though they are feeling better. Reports have noted male convalescent patients infecting their wives via sex even at 7 weeks. Likewise, some reports note women infecting their husbands after recovery and evidence supports lingering virus in vaginal mucus which could suggest similar immune privilege in ovaries as exists in testes. Part of the sexual mode of transmission can be understood by the cultural expectations where women are supposed to accommodate the desires of their husbands and their cultural beliefs often overstep logic and warnings from healthcare workers. Collective feelings about using condoms in parts of Africa is that to do so is a "dirty" way of having sex and men are noted to avoid using them which has also led to the spread of other diseases like HIV (Ebola Deeply, 2015). One report recorded results of virus isolation from a convalescent patient from a semen sample at 82 days. The virus that infected this patient had passaged through at least three other human patients before infecting that patient (Rodriguez et al., 1999). It is known that lab research with animals presents the evidence that with each passage of the virus through another host, the virus gains virulence and other characteristics that lead to higher titers, shorter incubation periods, and more severe symptoms. Often, certain viral aspects evolve while others devolve so a mutation allowing more infectivity may also cause the virus to be less fatal (Ryabchikova & Price 2004). In the same report, Virus was isolated from other mucous membranes (conjunctival, rectal, and vaginal mucosa) up to 33 days (Rodriguez et al., 1999). When filoviruses were first seen in Marburg Germany, the initial protocol was to have patients abstain from sex for a period of one year. A patient during another filovirus outbreak; that of Marburg, developed Uveitis 2 months after recovery from this disease. Uveitis is an inflammation of tissues inside of the eyes that involve the colored tissue of the eyes and those tissues attached making up the uveal tract. In this patient, virus was successfully cultured from the aqueous fluid of the eye, noting another point for consideration; someone recovering from Ebola or other filoviruses should avoid ocular surgery to prevent possible exposure to others during this surgery (Kuhn & Calisher, 2008; Howard, 2005; King et al., 2014; Lupi & Tyring, 2003).

Pregnant women frequently abort their pregnancy as noted in the previous section, and it is of note that pregnant women in general, with an altered immune system may be more susceptible to fatal infections with Ebola and other filoviruses. There are clinical observations indicating a high rate of death in children of infected mothers whether that is due to breastfeeding, which is widely known to contain virus, or through other care methods, close contact, or by secondary incidences that arise from being orphaned by the death of the parents. It is also notable that there are no reports as of this writing that conclude fetal or newborn survival when infected with Ebola (Baggi et al., 2014). Many references mention sharing a bed or room with an infected Ebola patient was the source of infection for a contact, which suggests aerogenic transmission although no specific contact is mentioned in any of those references (Lupi & Tyring, 2003; Reuters, 2014; Stern, 2014).

Immune Privileged Regions in the Body

Immune Privileged Regions of the body have been studied since the 1940s when Peter Medawar first used the term to describe the lack of and differences in immune responses with regard to transplanting of tissues. The similarities in the few immune privileged regions in the body are that they have barriers or separations from the blood system and mechanisms that prohibit innate and adaptive immune responses. These regions are in the testes, the eyes, the Central Nervous System (CNS), and the amniotic sac that holds amniotic fluid and a fetus during pregnancy. Immune privileged regions are limited in their ability to drain lymph which is a large part of the immune system's ability to clear pathogens. These sites also have cells that function to inhibit inflammation and immune reactions in those regions (Tafilaku, 2013, Winnall et al., 2014).

Regarding Ebola, these are the very same regions noted in the recent literature which when tested for virus even weeks into convalescence result in a positive test for live virus as mentioned earlier. This means that long after blood tests are negative for Ebola, fluids from these immune privileged regions retain the virus.

The testes have a barrier, a blood-testes barrier, which might be observed in ways similar to the blood-brain barrier that disallows certain substances like drugs from passing into the brain. In the testes, this is to prevent the body from identifying sperm as foreign material which would result in an immune attack on the sperm. This protects the sperm but also prevents immune access to virus that is allowed to persist in the testes which makes seminal fluid a high risk body fluid for as long as 89 days. Studies have shown that another virus, the HIV virus, can effectively persist in the testes (Tafilaku, 2013, Winnall et al., 2014).

In the eye, Anterior Chamber Associated Immune Deviation (ACAID) has been described for immune privilege in numerous studies. This immune deviation explains the observations of Ebola virus being found in the aqueous humor when a paracentesis is performed on convalescent Ebola patients in attempts to lower dangerously high intra-ocular pressure that is often seen along with inflammatory conditions like uveitis that result in closure of the drainage angle of the eye. Interestingly, this would not entirely explain how uveitis would be initiated. The sub-retinal space, located between the retinal pigment epithelium (RPE) and the photoreceptor cells is created by a barrier on the outer side of the RPE and the inner side of the space that is created by the positioning of the Muller cells in the adjacent retinal layer. These form a barrier that separates the space between from the body's blood supply. Findings by Anand et al. (2001) in their research of the sub-retinal space helped to illuminate the similar immune privilege characteristics and generation of immunosuppressive cells, making this space and possibly also the vitreous cavity containing the vitreous humor notable areas for observation of virus preservation following convalescence.

The Central Nervous System (CNS) has its own system utilizing the spine and spinal fluid which is known to be an immune privileged site.

Some kinds of tumors create acquired immune privilege that operates much like the immune privileged regions and therefore should be considered as another place where virus might hide to evade the immune system (Tafilaku, 2013).

Personal Protective Equipment

At the time of this writing, the required minimal PPE is being debated by the most involved international stakeholders for this outbreak, including but not limited to CDC, WHO, Médecins Sans Frontières (MSF), UNICEF, and CIDRAP. The level of protection is nonetheless to be based on degree of exposure expected. If one is dealing with a minimally symptomatic patient who is not coughing, vomiting or having diarrhea, or otherwise creating aerosols, the recommendations are more relaxed and include goggles, masks (N95 masks, PAPR, HEPA or N100 masks), gloves and suits to protect garments worn against the skin (partial protective clothing). It is notable that the PAPR respirators are considerably more expensive, more difficult to breathe and work in and have been reported to coincide with higher incidence of needle-stick injuries. N-95 masks will not allow a complete seal on bearded faces and could pose risks. In situations where either the patients or a cleaning task are expected to produce aerosols of infectious materials, the recommendations include overalls and coveralls that are especially resistant to liquid or fluid penetration, splash/ waterproof aprons, rubber boots, nitrile gloves covered by heavy duty gloves (like those used in household cleaning tasks), liquid/ fluid proof head coverings that drape over coveralls (or a full-length jumpsuit), with full face barrier and a respirator with an APF (assigned protection factor) of at least 50. This level of protection in a respirator would be equivalent to either a full-face-piece, air-purifying (negative-pressure) respirator or a half-face-piece "powered air purifying respirators" PAPR (positive-pressure) (Brosseau & Jones, 2014; UNICEF, 2014 Kuhn & Calisher, 2008; Borio et al, 2002).

Dexterity and the ability to perform certain tasks important to emergency care like being able to feel a pulse through the gloves has been noted to be diminished by the thicker gloves that are often used in chemical protection suits. The ability to effectively communicate with team members through head coverings has been an issue with certain PPE suits as well as diminished visual field (Coates, Jundi & James, 2000).

Gloves are the first thing we think of in terms of barrier nursing along with goggles and masks. Many different kinds of gloves are available and they all have their pros and cons. With treatment of Ebola patients in mind, the need to double glove, and the environments and needs for dexterity come to the forefront. Temperature of a person's hands inside of gloves has been shown to reduce the "breakthrough time" (referring to the time before a glove becomes permeable) which increases permeability and thus, potential for exposure to not only the pathogens, but also chemicals and other substances being handled. It has been observed that many health facilities and other companies that use gloves in their work are switching from latex to nitrile gloves due to the allergy potential of the rubber latex and also for performance. Even with the improved performance of better glove material, gloves should be changed regularly and between patients, and hands should be washed between glove changes (Korinth, et al., 2007).

PPE should be chosen based on the needs of the users and the facility's budget as well as the level of protection required to preserve the safety of the healthcare worker while allowing optimal performance. Current recommendations agreed upon by many global agencies that are involved with treatment of Ebola patients include those noted above (full-head covering with build in face shield that extends over shoulders, worn over a full length jumpsuit or similar with long sleeves that can be overlapped with 2 pairs of gloves, preferable an inner nitrile pair and an outer thicker, more durable glove) as well as a heavy waterproof apron, waterproof boots, and shoe coverings. This kind of PPE has been repeatedly difficult to work in for long periods and can contribute to fatigue and exhaustion of the healthcare worker as well as an increase in incidence of mistakes in patient care and accidents. The recommendations for time to work in this level of PPE in hot humid environments like West Africa are 40 minutes. This time could be increased for air-conditioned environments but the consideration is still present for accurately completing necessary tasks while in PPE. Using a buddy-system is arguably the safest way to do-doff and to work in PPE and also for disinfecting the PPE before it is removed and either safely discarded or disinfected for reuse (Bhadelia, 2014).

A glove design was developed several years ago by the French company, Hutchinson Sante, SNC, called G-VIR which is equivalent in thickness to double gloving with regular rubber or nitrile gloves. Those who were asked to try this glove design reported similar comfort and dexterity as they observed with double-gloving. The G-VIR gloves were deemed to be an improvement in high-risk situations where perforations via contaminated sharps were more probable because of the design which included an antimicrobial substance in a middle space between other layers of the glove material (dodecyl-dimethyl ammonium chloride, benzalconium chloride, and chlorhexidine digluconate with polyethylene glycol). The glove material itself is described as a synthetic thermoplastic elastomer (Caillot & Voiglio, 2008).

Nurses make up the largest group of healthcare workers and due to the nature of their work; they are more vulnerable to occupational exposures to pathogens in general. Studies examining compliance with procedures relating to safety while treating infectious patients (including reporting exposures) found that there is a significant number of nurses who fail to comply with those safety protocols for a variety of reasons, but most often, they claimed to be too busy or had fear of repercussions for not following a particular protocol to report the exposure. Considering Ebola, non-compliance with safety procedures, protocol and reporting of exposures could endanger not only those nurses who did so, but also others with subsequent exposures to those nurses (Efstathiou, et al., 2013).

General practitioners were also found to cut corners on safety-related protocols in studies even though they noted that they were familiar with the right way to perform. Those parts skipped were related to sterilization and disinfection such as washing hands between patients, wearing gloves for suturing or otherwise treating wounds, giving injections and even *fitting intrauterine devices* (emphasis added) except when driven by pressure from patients, health inspections, and threats of legal action (Gignon, et al., 2012).

Still other studies highlight the need to perform all patient care while observing universal precautions which are often not fully complied with. Those studies reveal statistics on exposures, sharps injuries, infecting patients, and other incidents where no gloves were being worn, no mask, goggles, or other precautions which were standard protocol (Sencan, et al., 2004; Efstathiou, et al., 2011; Amoran & Onweibe, 2013). These studies drive home the need to not only have adequate PPE but also to follow safety procedures and protocols closely.

Those working with and around Ebola patients must be trained in the donning, doffing (removal) and use of the various PPE as well as virus theory pertaining to how virus can infect humans. It is notable that the healthcare workers infected outside of Africa in Spain and in Texas, USA were reportedly infected while removing their PPE and it is probable to think that is also a factor in how healthcare workers become infected in Africa. In tropical Africa, where the heat and the humidity are high, workers cannot stay in the PPE for more than 30-40 minutes because it causes them to sweat and lose fluids and electrolytes more rapidly leading to dehydration and also leads to fatigue which accounts for accidents in numerous reports that study healthcare worker exposures and accidents. People wearing the PPE suits report that doing the most minor tasks result in profuse sweating inside the suits and they say sweat will often run down their faces. With this kind of situation, a person may reach to wipe the sweat and incidentally infect themselves (Brosseau & Jones, 2014; UNICEF, 2014; Young, 2007).

The behaviors of those wearing the PPE could impact their individual exposure probability. When people are required to work in the PPE much longer than the recommended time in such uncomfortable environments, they may be tempted to loosen or partially remove the garments which could allow exposures to occur (Chang, et al., 2007). Photos displayed in some of the early accounts of the outbreak revealed health care workers doing just that; rolling up sleeves while mopping floors, and wearing the jumpsuit unzipped partially.

Thoughts about which of these necessary materials might be related to cost, and one person's gear might cost $100 US or more. Any parts of the PPE that can be disinfected and washed using a chlorine solution is done, but if there is tearing or other breach of the garment's protection, it must be disposed of – incinerated, for the protection of those who wear these garments in attempts to slow and finally stop this outbreak.

One might suspect that conditions in developed countries with temperature controlled and pressurized facilities should be able to opt for more comfortable PPE and equipment. Use of negative pressure tents around patient beds and other sophisticated equipment could lessen the amount of PPE needed by the care givers as could the use of rooms equipped with telemedicine equipment where the care can be done robotically using monitors and related equipment. There is a consensus among groups discussing this topic in social media that there is a need for improvements in this area.

It is important for healthcare workers in every environment to learn and practice the proper techniques for putting on and removing their PPE. The WHO has brochures with pictures detailing the method they use and suggest having a buddy-system or at least an observer to be certain the donning and doffing of the PPE is accurate and that there are no rips or other penetrations in the protection. University of Texas Medical Branch has a document that details reasonable and useful PPE protocol which also adds the importance of removing jewelry, watches, pagers, phones, etc. from the persons to be entering a room with those suspected of a high containment disease (UTMB, 2013). It is even more important to learn and practice removal of the PPE, especially noting the case in Spain, as well as in the US, where the observation is that the women became infected while removing their PPE as noted above.

There has been criticism visible on a variety of social online groups that were based on the purchase of and assumed stock-piling of PPE components after two US nurses became infected. A report by Swaminathen, et al., 2007 that examined response to SARS in hospitals at that time revealed that in order to provide care to the range of expected cases (57,900 to 148,000), hospitals would need between 1,123,260 and 3,714,800 complete PPE sets. By comparison, even though Ebola has not proven to be airborne like SARS, caution has dictated the need for respiratory protection as noted elsewhere in this text, as well as the full PPE set of garments which must be removed at intervals and replaced with new sets each time a healthcare worker tends to a patient or cleans a patient room. This study justifies the purchasing of large numbers of PPE sets considering the projections that were being published by the CDC and WHO for new patient infections.

Disinfection and Decontamination

The use of sodium hypochlorite or household bleach is a mainstay in international response units that respond to Ebola and other hemorrhagic fever outbreaks. Ordinary household bleach (Clorox) has a 5.0% chlorine concentration. This disinfectant solution inactivates and disinfects enveloped viruses such as the Ebola virus and is inexpensive and relatively easy to mix, but should be done in a well-ventilated area or outdoors. A 1:10 mixture makes a 0.5% solution and can be made with any container by filling it once with the bleach, pouring that into a larger vessel, and then filling and pouring nine more times with water. Once this mixture is made, one can make a 0.05% solution by filling the same container once with this mixture and pouring that into a new vessel and then adding nine more containers-full of water to that. These solutions become inactive after 24 hours as the chlorine evaporates out of the solution over time. If the smell of chlorine is no longer present, discard the solution and make more (WHO, 2014).

The 0.5% or 1:10 solution is used for patient excreta on reusable surfaces and also on deceased bodies and can irritate skin, should be kept away from mucous membranes, and used with protective equipment in place. The weaker, 0.05% 1:100 solution is used for patient bedding and clothing, for surfaces, instruments and re-usable PPE before laundering, rinsing gloves between contact with each patient, rinsing gloves, apron, and boots before leaving the patient's room, and disinfecting contaminated waste for disposal. In the makeshift Ebola centers, healthcare workers fill containers that have plastic spigots on them with the 0.05% solution for ease of use, but a system can be constructed similar to those used on marine vessels and in other instances which employ a foot-operated valve to keep soiled hands off of the spigot (WHO, 2014).

Burial of deceased patients should be swift and with as little contact as possible while observing strict barrier isolation methods. Bodies should be disinfected thoroughly with the 0.5% bleach solution (King et al., 2014; WHO, 2014).

WHO has created an extensive and easy to read PDF document about disinfection and reuse of supplies that can be read for more extensive information. The link to the document can be found in the references section at the end of this writing.

There are additional household cleaners that can be effective including vinegar solutions. Vinegar and detergents like bar soap and laundry or dish detergents are effective on the lipid envelope of viruses and can be less caustic than bleach, or used where bleach allergies or sensitivities are concerned and cost is an issue (Jane et al., 2010).

Documentation of clinical data during Ebola outbreaks is important for all clinicians who are learning to treat and care for patients; those who are epidemiologists studying how the outbreaks begin and progress; for those researching preventative, prophylactic, and treatment therapies; and to others who work with disinfection and other protective measures for infectious diseases. There is not a complete source of clinical data from past Ebola outbreaks or all who are interested to study. It has been challenging for medical workers who treat Ebola patients in Africa to document every sign, symptom, and in-depth histories for each patient in order to provide a good understanding into how they were exposed, when and where and who they may have exposed for a number of reasons. Some of the reasons could be restrictions of being in PPE, the sheer number of patients encountered each day not allowing ample time for documentation and thus only hurried documentation of case information or none at all. Data that is documented has been destroyed after having been contaminated, or after attempts to decontaminate the chart or other means of documentation with bleach solutions. Numerous methods of approaching documentation have been tried and suggested but the most popular method among health care workers has been the use of two people where both are in PPE and one performs needed care while the other does the documentation. Dictating "over the fence" was also a popular option where the treating worker could dictate to another who was outside of the hot zone and who could safely document without fear of contamination of the chart (or electronic device being used if that was the case). Where reliable electricity was available, many health care workers liked the idea of using a personal electronic device like an iPad that was enclosed in a rugged waterproof (and thus easy to decontaminate) case (Buhler, et al., 2014).

Disposal of contaminated disposable materials requires decontamination with the 0.05% bleach solution after which they can be incinerated. In Africa, disposable contaminated materials are burned in metal barrels where the fire is tended to until everything has turned into ashes (WHO, 2014). In the US, the protocol is not that easy. Hospital medical waste is regulated in terms of biohazards and relating to either sharps or saturated medical waste. Anything that has blood or body fluids or tissue, etc. on it that is potentially absorbent is placed in red biohazard bags, labeled appropriately and stored for a short period of time before it is collected by companies that specialize in final disposal of the waste. Likewise, sharps and anything that is not absorbent is placed into a red plastic receptacle which is closed when nearly full and disposed of via professional biomedical waste companies. Because the US Department of Transportation makes the guidelines for transport of this biomedical waste and they classify Ebola as a "Category A Agent" meaning it is potentially life threatening, they require special packaging of the waste and HAZMAT (Hazardous Materials) training for those employees transporting it. Alternatively, the waste could be decontaminated. Some hospitals have the ability to steam autoclave the materials, but this is cost-preventative for most hospitals. As of this writing, it is noted that the CDC hopes to augment the rules to allow for rules about this sort of waste to be more allowing of care to prevent hospitals from having to turn away potential patients in case they might not be able to dispose of the waste (Steenhuysen, 2014).

Wipes

Traditional wipes like the Lysol and Clorox brands make note to be mostly effective against certain other enveloped viruses. Kodan wipes made by the German company Schulke are advertised to kill enveloped viruses in 30 seconds. Clinell Universal Sanitizing Wipes advertise efficacy even on soiled hands and equipment and are effective at killing enveloped viruses in 60 seconds. There are a wide variety of bleach-containing wipes marketed for healthcare use which would be useful for unsoiled surface cleaning.

UV Exposure

South Carolina doctor, Jeffery L. Deal, has gone to Liberia with his devices called TRU-D SmartUVC which are portable disinfection devices that use UVC light wavelengths as opposed to less effective UVA or UVB to inactivate RNA viruses. He notes that his method for disinfecting patient areas can inactivate the viruses by disrupting the structure of the viruses making them unable to replicate. Before the robotic devices can be deployed in a room, all surfaces have to be exposed, all drawers opened and all disposable or washable bedding and the like must be removed. Anything soiled with organic matter must be cleaned prior as the virus can remain infective and avoid deactivation while protected by organic material (Truscott & Friedman, 2014). Once prepared, the robots are remotely activated and rooms are sealed so no one can enter until the process is finished. Used as described, although maybe not practical in areas with little or no access to electricity, the makers claim the process to be 99.9 percent effective at disinfection (Fox News, 2014).

Heat

Heating as in cooking of cooking foods that are suspect to be harboring the Ebola virus, should be done so to at least 60°C or 140°F for between 30-60 minutes erring on the high side for caution, or boiling for 5 minutes at a full rolling boil (Public Health Agency of Canada, 2014). These recommendations, as noted earlier in the text, are not meant for food or meat; they are meant for instruments, utensils, and other small reusable items. Foods and in particular meats, suspected to carry Ebola virus should be brought to an internal temperature of 60°C or 140°F and held there for 60 minutes before eating if they must be eaten. The consumption of bush meat is covered in the section on Culture.

Peroxide Fogging

The company Med Effects is currently working with the Nigerian and Liberian Ministries of Health to combat Ebola with their Sanosil Halo Fogger system which uses a peroxide based substance to fog patient areas which inactivate the viruses and other pathogens including fungal and bacterial pathogens which might be concurrently present (Personal Communication, September 18, 2014).

Electrolyzed water/ Hypochlorous Acid

A company called Viking Pure has developed a series of machines that uses an electric source, water and salt to create hypochlorous acid which they have tested on many bacteria and viruses and found it to effectively kill all of them in under 60 seconds, often in under 30 seconds. Though the company has not tested it on Ebola viruses due to the need for a level 4 facility to do so, they did test it on other comparable enveloped as well as non-enveloped viruses. The solution could be made onsite at hospitals and treatment facilities with power and water supplies and it could provide an alternative disinfecting method where chlorine bleach was not desired because of the respiratory irritation caused by fumes it leaves behind. Unlike chlorine bleach solution, the hypochlorous acid solution made by this machine is not toxic to humans or animals but still will kill viruses and bacteria and has no residual odor. Parasites and other single-celled pathogens are not affected by the solution either. The company estimates that costs to make the solution are about 2 cents per gallon on average. Hypochlorous acid could be substituted in the disinfecting protocols where ever chlorine bleach solution or other chemical and often toxic disinfection solutions are noted (Dimmit, 2014; Personal communication with Wesley Rose January 7, 2015).

Protective Clothing Patient Bedding and Clothing

Laundry for PPE should be kept in special areas for this purpose and soaked at least 30 minutes in 0.05% bleach solution, being certain all parts are completely submerged. PPE is then transferred to bin of soapy water and then articles are left to soak overnight in the soapy water after which, stains can be scrubbed away. Once clean, PPE can be rinsed and line-dried allowing sun exposure is additive. Ironing can be used but is not necessary (WHO, 2014).

Additional procedures for mattresses and plastic sheeting used to protect mattresses can be read in the WHO guidelines which can be found in the references section.

Patient Excretions

Patient urine, stool, sputum, blood and any objects that make contact with patients or their body fluids such as lab equipment should be disinfected with 0.5% or 1:10 sodium hypochlorite solution before disposal or other sterilization methods. Disposable supplies, gauze, or other absorbent materials should also be disinfected and/or incinerated on site to prevent accidental exposures by those handling these (King et al., 2014; WHO, 2014).

Instruments (Adapted from the WHO Guidelines)

According to the WHO guidelines, 70% isopropyl alcohol (rubbing alcohol) can be used to disinfect stethoscopes and thermometers using a saturated cloth that completely covers the item with contact to all surfaces for 30 seconds, followed by air-drying on disinfected or sterile surface. The cloth is then discarded. Using the 0.05% bleach solution, the recommendation is to use a clean disposable cloth dipped into the bleach solution until saturated and then wiping of the items with the cloth. Additionally, thermometers can be left to soak submerged in the solution for 10 minutes but stethoscopes should be wiped and not submerged.

Basins used for bed-pans should be covered with the 0.5% bleach solution then emptied into isolated toilets or latrines, followed by soap and water cleaning which is also poured into the isolated latrine, and then filled with a rinse with the 0.05% bleach solution and allowed to air dry.

Patient eating utensils can be washed with the 0.05% bleach solution

Walls and floors can be sprayed with the 0.05% bleach solution and then wiped using cloths or a clean mop that is saturated with the same solution. If there is visible soil remaining, wash with soap and water.

Fluid Spills (Adapted from WHO Guidelines)

Spills of blood or other body fluids or vomit, feces, other excretions can be handled with a bucket filled with the 0.05% bleach solution. Dense spills should use the 0.5% first to saturate the material. The procedure should involve the use of a cup to carefully pour small amounts of the solution onto the spill to avoid splashing or aerosolization of the material being cleaned. Let the spill soak in the solution for at least 15 minutes before wiping up with soaked cloths, always using PPE. Discard cloths as infectious waste and finish by washing with soap and water.

Past Outbreaks

There have been 28 outbreaks of Ebola virus disease since it was first seen in Zaire in 1975-76 (29 if we look at the new Democratic Republic of the Congo outbreak as a separate outbreak, which officials there claim it to be). This number is not including those exposures in laboratories where research with viruses was being conducted. For these "Special Pathogens" an outbreak can be just one person becoming ill from an Ebola virus. There are numerous sources that investigate the aspects of each outbreak and give the minute details that are known about each so there is no need to replicate those here (CDC, 2014; Kuhn & Calisher, 2008).

Outbreaks of Ebola had before been controlled and eventually contained through the practices of barrier nursing, the treatment of patient excreta with formaldehyde and hypochlorite, focused attention on use and removal of PPE, disposal/decontamination/sterilization of contaminated materials, treatment and burial of deceased, and the institution of community awareness, making particular awareness of burial practices. In Africa, indigenous as well as Muslim and other religions practice rituals that involve washing or cleansing of the body that always has the propensity of infecting all of those who attend (Kuhn & Calisher, 2008; Howard, 2005; Haglage, 2014; Anderson, 2014).

Initial gains won by the virus were due to lax barrier methods; healthcare workers did not don their personal protective equipment, or they did not do it as prescribed, for a variety of reasons such as the idea that the patients they were working with were not suspected to be infected with Ebola, they dropped their guard to save face when a patient presented as fearful of the appearance of the PPE, or the heat was too overwhelming that they decided to loosen the restriction of those garments a bit (Kuhn & Calisher, 2008; Pattyn, 1978). Additional issues could be possible where health care workers had to deal with combative patients that compromised their PPE barriers, but there is little written to that end.

Reservoirs

After the 1975 identification of Ebola viruses, a researcher, Bruce Johnson, and his colleagues painstakingly collected hundreds of animals (monkeys and other species) looking for a potential reservoir. A reservoir is an animal that can have the virus circulating in their bodies and shed virus through saliva, urine, feces, or blood and never be sick from the presence of virus – asymptomatic. All of the sampling of the animals done by Johnson and his team was inconclusive but they did note some 26% of peri-domestic guinea pigs in Tandala region were antibody-positive although none were connected by any means to human involvement. They may have been an incidental host of virus without being a true reservoir (Howard, 2005).

Much has been researched about potential reservoirs since the appearance of filoviruses more than forty years ago. Some of those studies revealed additional aspects of the disease processes and are covered in other sections of this writing. In 2005 Leroy et al. found antibodies against Ebola in three species of fruit bats, which means that those bats were infected, went through a period of virus replication and survived the infection. One particular species of fruit bat found in West Africa was found to be a key reservoir for the Marburg filovirus species because it not only had antibodies, but researchers were able to isolate Marburg virus from its blood. Bats of various species are an important piece to the ecology and epidemiology of Ebola and other filoviruses, but as of this writing, no animal has been named as the main reservoir (Olival & Hayman, 2014; Biek, et al., 2006; Haglage, 2014).

A group of researchers studied the anthropological aspects of the disease at the origin of this outbreak in Guinea where many early reports said that a 2 year old child was the index patient and that he was infected by bush meat. This team was able to come to other conclusions after speaking with many people in the same village and also gathering data and testing local insectivorous bats for evidence of virus. Although none of the samples they collected yielded a positive test result for either virus or immune cells that would be indicative of an Ebola infection, the researchers feel that the presence of the species of bats that they found and the anthropological evidence is supportive of a theory that includes insectivorous bats and an alternate mode of initial infection of the index patient. They concluded that the index patient might instead have been infected while playing with the bats or otherwise exposed to the virus because of the bats (possibly feces or excretions, or other) which were largely insectivorous bats (Saez, 2014). It is easy to understand that virus is not always present in the animals which are presumed to be the reservoirs of the disease in nature, just as not all bats (foxes, skunks, etc.) have rabies. It is possible that the particular bats that are involved in the transmission are intermittently infected and have immune systems which are either capable of eliminating the virus very early, rendering it ineffective of killing or otherwise causing symptoms, or that the antibodies they manufacture in combating the infection are not residual, but as of this writing there are no publications that give any of this detail. There is however a publication that links some interesting evolutionary theories regarding flight, metabolism and other factors to the ability of many bat species to endure viral presence of numerous virus species without becoming sick. The pertinent information from this study (Zhang, et al., 2012) can be found in the later chapter on *Ebola Ecology, Bats, Pigs, and Arthropods.*

It is worth mentioning that the information below about dogs and their presence in Ebola-outbreak areas, their consumption of dead animals, and known infected material such as vomit from infected people while maintaining an asymptomatic status is suggestive of reservoir qualities. More research should be done to determine the possibility of dogs being considered potential reservoirs for Ebola viruses if nothing more than an incidental or secondary player to that light.

Additional discussion of asymptomatic carriers of Ebola is ahead in a separate section. Some of the information, especially that relating to the discovery of antibodies in guinea pigs, rodents and dogs, is important to the subject of reservoirs.

Some 2014 Data and Information

First Case and Contacts

The first case is presumptive to have been a 2-year-old child who became ill suddenly and then died in Meliandou in Guéckédou prefecture of Guinea on December 6, 2013. It remains unclear as to how the child was exposed, but some presume scenarios may be where the mother had been preparing a piece of bush meat where the child was able to touch and ingest that or some liquid associated with it. The child then infected the mother, sibling, a midwife, the grandmother, and one other and then the virus spread through healthcare workers because they had never suspected Ebola and therefore took no precautions against the virus. A more recent report published in December of 2014 makes connections about insectivorous bats being involved in the index case exposure as noted above (Saez, 2014). It would not be unrealistic to think that the mother of the child was the index patient who transmitted the virus to the child via breast milk. An infection in a young child with a naïve immune system might cause the child to succumb faster than an adult with a more robust immune system. There have been several discussions that sought to recreate a different version of the scenario leading up to the infection of the index patient which involved children playing around a hollow tree that was known to be a habitat for insectivorous bats (those that eat insects like mosquitoes) but the documentation was flawed in that all of the assumptions made were contradicted by the lack of supporting positive data and lack of any virus in all bats that were caught and sampled in that area (Saez, et al., 2014). Cases mounted and it was not until over a month later that the suspicion of the unidentifiable hemorrhagic disease, often in concurrence with Cholera, was given attention for what it was and the proper diagnosis. On January 24, 2014 a doctor in Tekolo called his superiors reporting strange deaths occurring that looked like Cholera. Cholera patients would present with vomiting, diarrhea, and dehydration as the first few patients did, but additionally, they all had fevers and at least one was having nose bleeding (Stern, 2014; PBS, 2014; Baize et al., 2014).

Because the grandmother of the index patient traveled to Guéckédou seeking help from a friend who was a nurse, she carried the virus there. Her friend did not know how to help her and she went back to her home where she died. The nurse in Guéckédou became sick shortly after and sought help from his friend, a doctor, living in Macenta where he slept in a room with the doctor's son. He died the next day but somehow infected the doctor and the son, who both died, but not before transporting the disease to more areas. Before his passing, the doctor from Macenta traveled to Conakry looking for answers to the mysterious outbreak when he developed symptoms that resembled those he had seen, but died in-route. His death triggered a call to WHO and teams went to collect evidence but even three months into this outbreak nobody knew precisely what disease was killing patients because many of them also tested positive for Cholera. It is logical to ask about the transmission between the male nurse and his friend (the doctor) and the doctor's son; if sharing a room was the only exposure then this raises questions about the mode of transmission. Because Ebola was never seen in this region it was not suspected; rather a first thought was Lassa or Yellow Fever (different hemorrhagic fever viruses very common to the region). The overarching symptom was hiccups and that was what prompted a senior researcher at MSF to start treating this like Ebola and order those tests and it was now March 14, 2014 and on March 20 the Institut Pasteur in Paris, France declared samples positive for a filovirus, ZEBOV (Stern, 2014).

Progression of the Outbreak

By the time Guinea reported the first set of cases as Ebola, there were at least 49 cases reported and because this region did not believe Ebola could be the cause of the illnesses, many people did not seek hospital care or report the illnesses and their observations of sick loved ones entering hospitals and either coming out in body bags, or not coming out at all fed their fearful beliefs that the space-suit-wearing health workers were doing some heinous activities to their loved ones. People avoided going to facilities, they escaped to neighboring villages, sought out traditional healers and all the while, spread the disease further. Rumors mounted, which are discussed below, and fear spread, both of the disease and the fear of government mal-intent among others and the rumors were, just like Ebola, not confined to Guinea (Youde, 2014; Mark, 2014; Fox News, 2014).

The hiding of disease by the population at large made it appear that the outbreak was becoming manageable and right about the time that they were about to announce it to be over, an explosion of new cases and deaths appeared as people likely were no longer able to handle deaths of relatives and caring for the sick. Deaths took the bread winners from families, took caregivers and parents away leaving children orphaned (as well as stigmatized) because not even those people who knew the children wanted to take them in remembering that diseases are thought to be caused by evil and curses and the like. Some children battled the disease in isolation while holding onto the images of their parents only to be discharged and learn their parents are dead from the disease. Depression sets in for these children as they wonder where they will stay and how they will survive as they are at the same time grieving the loss of their parents (Youde, 2014; Chen & Kitamura, 2014; Mark, 2014).

By April 1, 2014 countries offering flights to the affected areas began to implement safeguards against allowing the spread to their countries and borders in surrounding countries began to close with checkpoints installed to delay movement and observe travelers from one country to another for fevers and signs of disease. Eventually, flights were cancelled until further notice, hoping the outbreak would find its end as others had in the past (Stern, 2014; PBS, 2014; Reuters, 2014).

Near the end of May, the last 'known' contacts of the last 'known' Ebola patient in Conakry were declared symptom-free for the incubation period of 21 days. They assumed that because no new cases were reported that there were no new cases because they assumed the local people understood the urgency and importance of contact tracing and the need for intact epidemiological studies to be certain about the status of the outbreak. In Guéckédou, medics were only following a few more contacts, watching for development of symptoms and were hopeful and the CDC began dismissing staff and preparing to hand over treatment centers solely to local medical staff. Stunningly, a patient came to the Conakry center May 27, 2014 followed by five more June 2 and more after that. Some patients had traveled over 100 miles to get there, leaving a potential path of contact exposure behind them and the same sharp rise in cases was observed in the other region (Stern, 2014; PBS, 2014; Reuters, 2014).

As the outbreak gained momentum and more cases were found in additional regions, local healthcare was not able to maintain care of cases and began turning patients away. Local clinics in affected regions as well as those who caught word of the outbreak closed their doors, knowing they were not trained or capable of safely caring for Ebola patients or possibly also not willing to take the risk. A hospital in Kenema, Sierra Leone that has treated Lassa, another hemorrhagic fever for 25 years or more closed down after losing staff members while battling the disease. Now that the hospital is closed and its key staff dead, Lassa season is approaching (November to April) and there is still no end to the Ebola outbreak in sight (Hayden, 2014). Because of the closures of regular medical clinics, numerous other people fell victim to Ebola that were never infected and never tested positive, because of the lack of care for maternity needs, malaria needs and other regular emergency care that had been in place. Reports of women going home to give birth after being turned away from hospitals for fear of the usually bloody deliveries died from complications in delivery (Millar, 2014; Reuters, 2014).

On May 26th, Sierra Leone confirmed the first Ebola death and then on July 25th, Nigeria registered one case of a Liberian-American man who traveled to Lagos to seek care. Nigeria reacted quickly and like other regions, they closed schools to prevent spread. Other regions, like those in Liberia where suspicion and lack of trust abounds, closed their schools after rumors circulated about health workers taking blood samples from the children were instead infecting the children with the deadly disease. At the time of this writing, Nigeria is watching the last of their contact traced individuals for symptoms and hoping for a declaration of being Ebola-free (Reuters, 2014; Stern, 2014).

On August 24th, DRC reported a separate outbreak in an isolated area of its northern Equateur Province. This outbreak is being treated as a separate outbreak as the sequencing of the virus from the DRC circulating virus has been called clearly different from that circulating in the other regions. Then on August 29th, Senegal reported a first case in their country (Reuters, 2014; International Society for Infectious Diseases, 2014; Sanchez, 2014).

In West Africa, Ebola virus disease was never a concern so presumed diagnoses of the first few dozen or more patients were thought to be anything from Cholera, which was very common, malaria, Yellow Fever, or Lassa fever (Stern, 2014; PBS, 2014). In filoviral disease, prostration (meaning the need to lay flat on the ground, bed etc. and loss of energy or desire to even sit up, weakness and exhaustion), lethargy, wasting (likely due to the associated loss of appetite and nausea upon ingestion of any substance), and diarrhea are usually more severe than those symptoms observed in patients with other viral hemorrhagic fever and in the 2014 outbreak, the hemorrhagic symptoms were not as prevalent as the aforementioned symptoms which explains the difficulty in recognizing the disease as Ebola in the earlier phases of this outbreak (International Society for Infectious Diseases, 2014 (174); Lupi & Tyring, 2003).

In mid-September, deaths of 12 including a doctor and three nurses in Ghana were reported to be from Cholera where some 117 cases occurred and no suspicion as of that report was noted to be relating those deaths to Ebola (Ghana Web, 2014).

Control of the outbreak with consideration of air travel and preventing pandemic spread has proved to be challenging with the widespread reporting in countries where news media had rarely ventured to report on African outbreaks. Because of the coverage of surveillance, people attempting to travel from outbreak affected regions to other countries are aware of methods used to prevent those suspected of infection from travel and even if they have no known exposures, fear of detainment and subsequent delay of travel and costs incurred for airfare lost pose a formidable reason to avert surveillance. A Liberian national did just that as he lied on an exit survey to make a flight to the U.S. in September. He knew he had been exposed to a dying victim right before his departure and his deceit led to a frustrating series of events inside of the U.S. which included the infection of at least one nurse who cared for him before he died of the disease in early October (Onishi, 2014).

The disease spread to Mali via a small child whose family recently died from the disease. Mali was declared Ebola-free in mid-January, 2015. Liberia's documented cases began to fall in number in late 2014. Sierra Leone was not so fortunate; after the disease found its way into Sierra Leone, it spread rapidly and as of this writing, continues to spread because of the same cultural practices and stigmas noted earlier in reference to Liberia (WHO, 2014; WHO, 2015).

Lack of Public Health Infrastructure

The World Health Organization has reported that the countries affected by Ebola, (Liberia, Sierra Leone, Guinea, Nigeria, DRC, Mali, and Senegal) among many others, about 25 to 40 percent of people lack access to safe, clean water, protected from outside contamination and in particular feces. About 17% of the populations in these countries have access to toilets and most people practice open defecation. Some homes may not even have access to soap. This percentage increases dramatically for the more rural areas away from what infrastructure the towns and cities provide. Reports note health centers treating Ebola patients might not have access to running water which makes washing and disinfecting more difficult, maybe impossible (Mis, 2014).

African Minister's Council on Water (AMCOW), executive secretary Bai-Mass Taal told reporters that in times before Ebola, some 65% of hospital beds were taken by those sick with water-borne illness traceable use of the local water to drink and for hygiene. AMCOW is a body of government ministers from 53 member states in Africa. This lack of infrastructure may delay treatment for some and could pose other threats from contamination even though virus could be diluted by the combining with water (Mis, 2014).

The hospitals and clinics in the same areas were poorly stocked with supplies prior to the outbreak and are in dire conditions without supplies being routed to them. This is especially true while borders are closed and road, as well as air travel is limited. A report from 2009 lists all of the known hospitals in all of Africa and there is a paucity of hospitals in the West African regions hardest hit in this outbreak (PBS, 2014; VICE News, 2014; Agenda for Environment and Responsible Development, 2009).

Rumors and Other Aspects That Prevent Control of the Outbreak

Numerous rumors began to spread in Liberia where civil war had created a rift between the people and the government that prevented trust and so the people were skeptical of what the government said about Ebola. Rumors were told about Ebola being a lie and that the government wanted to take the blood of the poor people (and possibly sell it) (PBS, 2014). President Olusegun Obasanjo of Nigeria, said in a public speech that the index patient in his country, "Patrick Sawyer, in a devilish connivance with some Liberian authorities, intentionally brought the disease to Nigeria" (Gbadamosi & Olukoya, 2014).

Following this distrust of government and officials, in Liberia, many people still verily believe that the outbreak is a lie started by government officials who hoped this sort of disease would distract the population away from a series of recent scandals, or for health officials to profit from money required for care of the sick. A man interviewed in Liberia told reporters that he and others there believe that Ebola is a terrible disease, but they all agree it is not in Liberia and that the story and drama was dreamed up by the government to "divert the Liberian's mind" (Mark, 2014).

There are rumors among the local populations in Liberia that in those Ebola tents, the MSF are collecting peoples' body parts or that they are taking their blood (Journeyman Pictures, 2014; VICE News, 2014). In an interview with people in a market selling various smoked and dried bush meats, the consensus was that the Liberian government was broke because they squandered money and that they conjured up the "Ebola scam" to coerce international communities to give them more money. They also believed the government had some mal-intent for telling the people not to eat bush meat.

Women were telling the reporters that they have been eating bush meat for centuries and have had no sicknesses so why should they go hungry now. They followed by saying Ebola was never seen in their country so they do not believe the warnings (VICE News, 2014; PBS, 2014).

Fear has been a continual roadblock to the successful control and cessation of this outbreak. Even in the beginning, as health workers moved in to set up tent hospitals and begin taking in patients, the fear, driven by rumors caused local populations of people to hide if they were sick, hide their loved ones and delay or never report dead or very sick people. Because of this fear, officials with international health organizations and missions believe a mere third of cases are reported, and they also say that they might have gotten control of the outbreak early on if fear had not driven the sick to flee, hide from others and spread the disease to neighboring towns. In mid-September, a group of 8 health officials and journalists have been killed due to this fear as they made attempts to educate villagers about the disease and try to prove that health care workers were there to help, not harm. This kind of attack on health care workers may prevent more volunteers from agreeing to go to their aid (Callemachi, 2014; Fox News, 2014).

In many of the affected regions there is little or no health infrastructure; the region of Kailahun has only four ambulances in a population of almost 500,000. Notable too, when the ambulance takes in a sick person that person's whole family will pile into the vehicle where in close quarters often become exposed to the virus on the ride to the hospital (Mark, 2012). In other areas of Liberia, medical workers use hearses in place of ambulances due to a shortage of vehicles for this purpose (PBS, 2014).

There continue to be reports of families quietly burying bodies without sanitary practices so they can continue to perform traditional burial rituals. These practices have added to the complexity of controlling and finally halting this outbreak. Recently, removing Ebola-infected dead bodies from clinics or even homes has been made illegal in some parts of West Africa to aid in stopping these rituals which have been documented to spread the disease to many other people. Even the threat of arrest has not stopped the practices though, and rather, has inspired even more covert actions such as changing death certificates to relay a cause of death other than Ebola. A particularly disturbing case was involving the death of a woman in Liberia where her relatives dressed her corpse and set her in a car between two other ladies making her appear alive so she could be driven to a site for ritual burial. This particular case exposed some 2000 or more people to the disease who are now being followed in quarantine (Tamba, 2014).

Also in Liberia, the government ruled against further cremation of dead bodies. This decision was made based on the actions such as those described in the last paragraph, where families hid their sick and or dead loved ones to avoid altered funeral rites and cremation of the bodies. The Liberian decision makers hope that by abolishing cremation requirements more of the sick will seek treatment and that fewer families will try to hide their dead and perform risky funeral rituals on those bodies, thereby perpetuating the spread of the disease (Harmon, 2014).

The complacency among populations in Africa as well as those in other countries is a prevailing cause for concern. In Africa, concerning Ebola virus, when the disease has gone away for a time period and becomes silent in the thoughts of the population, the practices of the people become more lax, hospital and clinic workers are not all adhering to universal precautions despite the numerous other infectious diseases present like HIV. Gloves get used again and again in the spirit of possibly protecting the healthcare worker, but if they read the manufacturer's documents about disposable gloves, they have a short usage span. Nitrile gloves have been the recommended best choice by many entities involved in actual healthcare because of durability and absence of the latex allergy issues. Aside of the materials, wearing any gloves too long will allow permeability to one extent of another so it is important to know the wear life of the particular gloves being used especially when working in environments that expose the wearer to Ebola viruses. CDC recommends 'heavy duty' gloves and nitrile gloves can suffice for the first layer of protection followed by a larger nitrile glove to allow for movement and prevention of constriction of movement and a third layer can be added using a larger glove, or for heavy cleaning purposes, those gloves used for household chemical cleaning can be employed atop the other two layers while keeping in mind, the relative time required to change gloves to prevent permeation by unwanted microbes. Another good indicator is color change; if gloves change color, they should be discarded and replaced. No matter which gloves are selected for use, they should be removed in a safe way to prevent contamination of skin during removal and hands should then be washed every time (CDC, 2014).

Notable Epidemiology/ Cases

Dr. Richard Sacra was working in a center for pregnant women where he delivered babies and gave maternal care during the 2014 outbreak. He was known to have written protocols for Ebola PPE and was wearing PPE despite his work not being conducted in an Ebola-specific hospital. Despite his attention to protocol for avoiding blood and body fluids, he became infected and had to be flown to a Nebraska containment hospital (Croteau, 2014; Weiss, 2014).

In a Medecins Sans Frontieres case management center in Foya, Liberia, an 11 year old boy named Mamadee was admitted on August 15th, 2014 but tested negative for Ebola. He stayed overnight in the center's guesthouse and planned to make the long trip back to his village the next morning but he developed symptoms overnight including nausea, fever, muscle pain, fatigue, abdominal pain, jaundice, and diarrhea. He tested positive for Malaria and doctors treated him for this. He began to feel better and regain energy, but doctors ran a second Ebola test where he tested positive on August 20th followed by yet another test a few days later which was also positive. Mamadee was admitted to the Ebola ward due to the positive tests, but he continued to thrive and had no more symptoms, as if the malaria possibly caused the initial symptoms (and possibly primed his immune system). By August 30, Mamadee was complaining of boredom and wanted to leave but another Ebola test was still positive noting the boy continued to shed virus even though he was Asymptomatic. While he remained in the ward without symptoms, his 14 year old sister Mayan was admitted and died within days. Mamadee was declared cured and free of disease/ virus on September 4, 2014 (MSF, 2014).

In late September, a nurse's assistant in Spain was diagnosed with Ebola after taking part in care of two Ebola patients and disinfection of rooms those patients died in. She claims she wore the recommended PPE but somehow still became infected. As of this writing, the actual route of exposure is unknown but it is speculated that it was as she took off her PPE. Additional comments are being made about the Spanish hospital using level 2 PPE which was not waterproof and that they were not provided respirators (Smith-Spark & Perez Maestro, 2014). Also in late September was the case mentioned above of the Liberian man who flew into Texas and later presented to a Texas hospital with initial symptoms of Ebola where there is ongoing debate about the sequence of events leading to his discharge and subsequent re-admission and isolation with Ebola. Issues being scrutinized in social media include those relating to misuse of antibiotics, inability to effectively communicate and question the patient about recent travel from outbreak affected countries, exposures of others, contamination of emergency vehicles and personnel among others (Onishi, 2014).

A nurse who was infected in the care of Mr. Duncan in Texas is undergoing isolation and treatment along with a close contact at the same hospital at the time of this writing. It is noted that her exposure was during removal of the PPE and Dr. Freiden, Director of CDC, remarked about the difficulty of removing respirators and other PPE safely as he revealed details about this patient (Cohen, Almasy & Yan, 2014).

In December, a four year old girl was observed caring for her mother in a Sierra Leone Ebola isolation ward. It is interesting that she was allowed to sleep next to her sick mother in this ward, but she never fell ill. It is unclear whether she was tested for Ebola, but after caring for her mother and essentially losing her mother and father to Ebola in the end, she never showed any symptoms of the disease. It is postulated that her father had been some sort of medicine man which would explain where Ebola made its way into her family as he likely was called upon to treat other Ebola victims with traditional healing methods when they would not trust clinics (Gentleman, 2014).

Asymptomatic Virus Shedding/ Carrying

A 1996 outbreak of Ebola in Gabon, where fatality rates ranged between 66% and 75%, revealed an interesting discovery; it was observed that at least 24 people who were in direct contact with materials from symptomatic patients or who cared for and lived with symptomatic patients never got sick themselves. Researchers obtained blood samples from these people several times during course of observations and tested for IgM and IgG antibodies as well as Ebola-specific RNA and cytokines. Their results revealed what they described as, "Asymptomatic and replicative Ebola infection in 7 of those people. The first samples taken from all of them had no antibodies which ruled out any prior exposures. Tests to determine presence of virus in a selection of these patients was done and they confirmed "transient virus replication" (in mononuclear cells) that lasted about 2 weeks. High concentrations of pro-inflammatory cells (cytokines) were found in samples taken about 1 week after the potential contact or exposure with infective source, but they were only present for 2-3 days. No T-cell derived cytokines or Ebola specific antigen were detected in asymptomatic patients during the entire study. Cytokines derived from T-cells are seen in cases that progress to fatal hemorrhagic disease. Testing of the white blood cells (where Ebola virus would replicate in the patient) in these asymptomatic patients all showed low-level viral load (Leroy et al., 2000). Another difference in immune response is notable between asymptomatic and symptomatic patients where those with no symptoms have IL-1B, IL-6, and TNF early on but none of the patients exhibiting symptoms had these mediators in their blood (Ryabchikova & Price, 2008).

Even in the first known outbreaks of Ebola in 1976-1979, WHO health workers observed people who appeared to have mild or no symptoms as well as those with fatal disease progressions in Sudan and Zaire. Unfortunately, none of those cases were sampled for virus or antibody testing; they were only observed for the incubation period. Likewise, in the Kikwit outbreak, DRC, testing revealed the suggestion of asymptomatic and mild cases alongside the serious and fatal cases (Leroy et al., 2000; Howard, 2005).

After a 1972 accidental injury/ infection of a doctor who performed an autopsy on what he thought was a yellow fever patient; where he got a fever, researchers tested the local population for antibodies and found a 7% seroprevalence for Ebola antibodies which indicated possible asymptomatic shedding (Howard, 2005).

In 1984-1985, a study revealed that 10% of 471 suspected Ebola cases (due to their contact with known cases) had antibodies to Ebola where the case fatality rate was only about 5%, suggesting that the virus causing the seroconversions belonged to neither of the known serotypes of the day, despite cross-reacting for reference strains in testing (Howard, 2005).

Studies in guinea pigs and mice are characterized by mild subclinical infections upon a first inoculation using a 'wild type' Ebola virus (one not used to inoculate other animals, which would then be cultured to grow new virus; each time this is done it is called a 'passage'). After serial passage of the virus the pathogenicity and lethality of that virus strain increases (Leroy et al., 2000).

In Liberia, there have been reports of dogs eating the dead bodies of Ebola victims that were either buried in shallow graves or not at all (Blake, 2014). This is an interesting point considering the community's collective set of beliefs about treatment of dead bodies and their rigid grasp of traditional burial practices. Some research into the phenomena of dogs near Ebola outbreaks and their propensity to play a role in the ongoing outbreak revealed at least one study that proves Ebola infection in dogs is possible and has been documented. In one report from 2005, researchers were interested in the role of dogs during past Ebola outbreaks so the samples blood from 439 dogs in Gabon in the region bordering DRC where outbreaks were reported between 2001-2002. They found between 8.9% and 31.8% seropositivity (presence of IgG) in the dogs, ranging based on the region where they were found and the highest percentages were where human Ebola cases were also reported. No Ebola antigen or nucleotide sequences were found in the samples, and they were unsuccessful in attempts to isolate virus in VeroE6 cells (the common cell culture used for Ebola virus isolation). In addition to making observations of these dogs, the researchers also interviewed dog owners locally and others who saw the dogs interacting with humans and living in the areas specified. What they learned was that these dogs were known to eat Ebola-infected dead animals, organs left over from animals killed in hunts, and even seen licking the vomit from Ebola-infected humans. None of the dogs had exhibited symptoms of illness despite their risky exposures but they may excrete virus for a short period after initial exposures via their blood, urine, feces, and saliva. In the study, it is also noted that goats and horses have been known to remain asymptomatic or to show only mild symptoms to Ebola infections (Allela et al., 2005).

A study of Non-Human Primates (NHP) in Gabon and Cameroon where researchers sampled over 400 (444) animals from 11 species, noting seropositive IgG rates ranging by species from 2.7% to 17.6%, the highest percentage was in chimpanzees. What this suggests is that chimpanzees are in continuous contact with the virus in their environment and live after being infected. It also suggests that asymptomatic or non-lethal cases of Ebola exist in NHP like it does in humans (Leroy et al., 2004).

Another outbreak of Ebola was when the Reston Ebola virus was first discovered, in a dramatic sequence of events involving the Reston Virginia Monkey House where a variety of NHPs were kept before sending them off to other labs for research. A disease spread through the air conditioning system and killed various monkeys in every room of the building due to the airborne nature of the virus. As dictated so fiercely in Richard Preston's Book about the Hot Zone, those involved, including researchers from USAMRIID (United States Army Medical Research Institute of Infectious Diseases) were astonished to learn that the causative agent was Ebola and after feverish urgent research, they were more astonished to find that this was a new strain that was not symptomatically affecting humans, although it did cause seroconversion in humans exposed, but it was lethal to NHPs. After this happened, a similar outbreak was observed in Siena, Italy with the same symptoms, notably high titer in respiratory secretions which signifies the transmission via air, but still no human illness, only seroconversions (Howard, 2005).

Some compelling research published near the end of the year 2014 about spread of various diseases among humans and animals shines light on another interesting phenomenon. A new concept of so called "Superspreaders" and also "Supershedders" where a percentage of the population in humans or various animals is responsible for more of the spread of illnesses than the larger percent of those populations. Interestingly, researchers doing this work found the percent of superspreaders in any population to be 20% for 80% of disease spread. This is the same concept presented in the Pareto Principle that is often referenced in business describing distribution of wealth and profits, but it applies to many other situations as well. In their work, researchers noted not only environmental situations such as employment creating optimal exposure environments for more spread, but also biological processes where the individuals had immune systems that would become accustomed to the pathogens and tolerant of high titers of those pathogens without a resultant illness or with only low-levels of illness which allowed them to spread the pathogens to others. Additionally, they found that there was a propensity for those spreading to shed much more virus or other pathogen; 100K pathogens from a superspreader vs. 100 pathogens from an average individual (human or animal). In addition to this immunological tolerance, there was a tendency for those spreading diseases to not fully clear the infection once symptoms were no longer present in those who developed symptoms (Reddy, 2014). This prolonged infection would allow the individuals to spread to others for a longer period. With Ebola specifically, noting the prolonged retention of the virus in certain body fluids, especially those which are from immune privileged sites, superspreaders and supershedders could be part of the underlying reason for the outbreak reaching proportions observed in 2014.

Recombination in Ebola Viruses

Recombination of viruses in the environment generally would require a single host to be infected with more than one lineage of a particular strain of virus, for example, a lineage of ZEBOV that has characteristics making it less virulent and another lineage of ZEBOV with characteristics making it more virulent. Recombination might yield novel progeny that have additional characteristics from each lineage that may circulate and become more prevalent due to positive selection of traits that allow the virus to continue to infect new hosts, become more stable in hosts and interim environments like on surfaces of in varying pH or temperatures (Cann, 2005; Wittmann et al., 2007).

Research studies have described the lineage of various EBOV species and outlined theories on their emergence based on virus spillover from one or more reservoir animals. Using genes from ZEBOV, a team was successful at demonstrating recombination between two distinct lineages, which they estimate, created the group of viruses that were responsible for the outbreaks in Gabon near the DRC border between 2001 and 2003. The researchers sequenced genes of ZEBOV from the carcasses of NHPs found between 2001 and 2006 and compared the major sequences which revealed substantial differences in the GP and NP genes at the nucleotide and amino acid levels. After looking closely at the sequences from all available human samples from the outbreaks occurring since 2001, they concluded that they were different than the sequences from all other earlier outbreaks in various regions of Africa between 1976 and 1997. Acknowledging the existence of apathogenic lineages of ZEBOV as suggested in the section here on Asymptomatic Disease, they explained that their data revealed existence of another ZEBOV lineage that is capable of infection and mortality in humans and animals which apparently arose in this small border region. They further suggest that this new group of viruses is migrating East based on observations of outbreak characteristics between 2001-2005. It is further suggested that there could be further recombination between live-attenuated virus strains and wild-type viruses that would result in menacing repercussions for public health (Wittmann et al., 2007).

It is notable that a study from 2011 reviewed the data from the work of Wittman et al. and noted that aside of this data, which was only based on two distinct genes; it has been proven that it is possible to have co-infection by multiple lineages or strains of filoviruses at the same time. Thusly, if samples are exhibiting multiple strains of filovirus, the PCR testing which involves amplification of the genomic regions can lead to the generation of artificially recombinant sequences making it necessary to perform additional testing to sort out the breakpoints (Han & Worobey, 2011).

Observations were made by a different team in 2000 that explain recombination like these may be due to positive selection that was driven by host immune pressure or even a change in the natural host animal allowing additional animals to carry the virus. These changes, at the cellular level exerted pressure on the NP gene which has protective effects for the viral genome (Leroy et al, 2002). The most recent research published openly by a team led by Pardis Sabeti included sequencing of all of the virus samples collected in the region where the outbreak began. Her team made inspiring progress even after losing several of their fellow researchers to the disease. Sabeti's research in 2012 in Nigeria found genetic similarities between Lassa and Ebola and she presumes that it is possible that Ebola was present in West Africa long before it was seen in this current outbreak and that is was misdiagnosed due to the similarities in symptoms (Gire et al., 2012; Gire et al., 2014). It is plausible to think that Ebola disease could be Lassa because locals are familiar with Lassa and they might not reach as far as to suspect Ebola. There is a saying, "If you hear hoof-beats, think horses rather than zebras" and Dr. C. J. Peters made the distinction in his book about Level 4 viruses, that in order to detect these viruses accurately one must always suspect those zebras; this holds especially true now as the global community works to hold back a pandemic of Ebola.

Ebola Ecology, Bats, Pigs and Arthropods

Atherstone, Roesel, and Grace (2014) mapped the geographic distributions of the bats which were reported in the literature to have been found positive for Ebola virus antigen, virus itself, or antibodies and they discovered an interesting pattern of overlapping distributions of those various bat species. The geographic coverage by all known bats to be positive for any of those tests span much of Sub-Saharan Africa, extending up into areas of Sudan, Ethiopia, and even as far as Yemen to the North and Mozambique to the south. Pinzon et al (2004) discovered a correlation between climate and outbreak incidence where their map images that predicted outbreak-prone areas overlapped areas where the 2014 outbreak occurred. Climate and rainfall effects on vegetation in the region are also notable in that they bare resemblance to those of Atherstone, Roesel, and Grace for their bat geography.

It is noteworthy that pigs have been observed to have concentrated illness in the lungs and respiratory tracts when infected with Ebola. When symptomatic, pigs are described as coughing forcefully, like a cannon (Atherstone, Roesel & Grace, 2014; Flohr, 2013; The PigSite, 2014). Pigs consistently replicated Ebola virus following a mucosal exposure, in their respiratory tracts, where they shed virus from their nasal mucosa up to 14 days, with observation of severe lung infection. Another observation was that of the infection of all susceptible pigs nearby that were inhabited with the infected animals, noting probable air-related transmission. The culminating observations are that pigs have been proven to transmit EBOV from infected pigs to naïve pigs in experiments which support the possibility of aerosol transmission by pigs (Infectious Diseases Society of America, 2011).

Research has proved that pigs are naturally infected with EBOV. When infected, pigs are mostly asymptomatic with REBOV and exhibit severe lung disease with ZEBOV. Outbreaks of porcine respiratory infections are easily misdiagnosed because like human diseases, porcine diseases have similarities in initial symptoms that mimic an array of other possible diagnoses. Observations made from African swine fever outbreaks in Uganda revealed that farmers still sold the infected pigs, ate meat from those pigs and sold pigs preferentially if they appeared sick to avoid waste of the pig's value. These kinds of practices would certainly amplify risks for Ebola in humans if it were present in farmed pigs (Atherstone, Roesel & grace, 2014).

The demand for pork meat across sub-Saharan Africa has risen over the last ten years as more farmers trade chicken and other animal farming for pig farming (Smallstarter Thinktank, 2013). Farming pigs allows a higher yield in less time and more money to the farmer in less time compared to farming of other species. Pigs can have over 8 piglets in a litter and take just 114-116 days for gestation (Haines, 2014) after which, the piglets can be weaned as early as 10 days although 3-5 weeks is considered to be better (The Pig Site, 2006a). So in roughly 4 months, maternal pigs can become pregnant again and have 8+ more piglets which in terms of farming for meat could be much more profitable than the breeding and husbandry of other species.

Pig meat is eaten for Christmas, Easter, and other special occasions in some African countries and is considered to be a luxury food by many. These holidays coincide with the relative times that outbreaks have occurred whether there is some connection or not, it is notable. The farming of pigs has become a popular means of income even to those who do not eat pork due to their religious beliefs like Muslim and Jewish populations because of the marketability of the meat to foreigners (Smallstarter Thinktank, 2013).

As mentioned in an earlier section on reservoirs, bats have been found to be competent reservoir animals for Ebola and other filoviruses. There are numerous studies reporting their search for the reservoir pointed to fruit bats. Lab research has been conducted and revealed that certain bat species were capable of supporting infections from Ebola and surviving through them while supporting virus replication to high titers. Testing of feces from those bats even at 21 days post infection revealed virus isolation (Howard, 2005; Kuhn & Calisher, 2008). So environments where bats roost can be contaminated with virus via feces and urine.

Epidemiological studies of past outbreaks sometimes found environmental aspects to be important because bats shared the space with humans either in their place of work, a cave, or in the forests where bats contaminated surfaces or food that humans ate, or hand contact with where fomite contamination was transferred to mucous membranes. Animals became infected similarly by sharing of the environment with bats (Atherstone, Roesel & grace, 2014). There are some 925 known species of bats, both insectivorous and frugivorous (eat fruit) but not many have been sampled for filovirus or IgG (Kuhn & Calisher, 2008).

Two species of bats in particular, Eidolon helvum (Straw-Colored Fruit Bat) and Hypsignathus monstrous (Hammer-headed Bat), have a very wide geographic range that covers all of the areas now affected by Ebola outbreaks over time. These species live in the canopies of tall trees in forests as well as in caves and can live 20 to 30 years. Other species that are known to have tested positive for virus isolation and or antibodies to Ebola are found in all parts of Sub-Saharan Africa with intersecting and convergent habitats. It is possible that more than one bat species are involved in some sort of sylvatic cycle where various bat species have particular important roles, which may at some point converge with incidental human and or animal exposures (Atherstone, Roesel & grace, 2014).

Several references identify these bats as being omnivorous (eating fruits, flowers and young leaves of plants) but the term, omnivorous, typically refers to animals which eat a meat protein and also plant-based foods but none of those references mentioned which protein was part of their diets to warrant classification as omnivorous rather than herbivorous. Here, one might assume that they also eat insects periodically and this is reasonable for their geographic distribution (African

Wildlife Foundation, 2014; Atherstone, Roesel & grace, 2014). These bats are also considered crepuscular and nocturnal so they might eat insects that are also. Some research reveals the following mosquito species that are crepuscular and nocturnal in the same geographic regions of Africa: Anopheles gambiae, Aedes, aegypti, Aedes albopictus, A. luteocephalus, A. rittatus, A. africanus, A. stegomyia, A. cumminsii (Aedimorpus subgroups), Culex quinquefasciatus, C. annulioris, Eretmapodites chrysogaster, E. quinquevittatus, Mansonia Africana, and M. uniformis. Some of these species are already considered to be important vectors of other diseases in Africa and globally. Bats in these regions would have a good supply of mosquitoes to feed on during the rainy seasons, but when dry season starts, mosquitoes are not as easily bred so their numbers are reduced dramatically. It is not clear what roles mosquitoes play or even if they do have a role in a sylvatic cycle with Ebola.

A study of evolutionary changes in many bats regarding their metabolism and how flight plays a role in capability of bats to endure presence of many species of viruses was conducted by Lin-Fa Wang and colleagues. They found some interesting differences in bat immune systems which could explain why they are capable of hosting various viruses without becoming ill from those infections. Bats are the only mammal capable of sustained flight. It is hypothesized that the genetic determinants that allowed the evolution of flight in bats also allowed evolution of their immune system to prevent DNA damage that would occur from this activity which creates an elevated metabolic rate and also a higher body temperature. Bats are known to carry many deadly diseases and live to spread them including but not limited to Nipah virus, Marburg, Hendra and SARS. It is probable that their sustained higher body temperatures do not allow the virus to replicate well, while other evolved aspects of their immune systems repair any damage viruses are able to do quickly which would allow a subclinical version of the infection to persist for some time period (Zhang, et al., 2012; Wynn & Wang, 2013).

Marburg virus was replicated in Aedes aegypti mosquitoes in one study which was not successfully replicated in subsequent studies. One study refers to use of REBOV in the same mosquitoes without success but suggested a different outcome could be possible using ZEBOV (Reiter et al., 1999; Swanepol et al., 1996). In the search for reservoirs and possible vectors in arthropods in outbreak regions of Africa, researchers collected some 35K+ insects and had no positive test results for virus isolation of Ebola or PCR but those collections were made from ground levels and it is notable that none of the specimens were collected from the canopies of the tall trees where bats roost. The collection of specimens was conducted about four months after the index patient was infected which could easily have missed the window of opportunity to find a positive result if the insects were only carrying infected blood while a migrating reservoir animal was present (Kuhn & Calisher, 2008). This lapse of time could have given ample time for the source of the virus to migrate from the area. Mosquito involvement during that time could have been transient, only becoming important as certain environmental aspects such as rainfall, coupled with fruiting of plants and trees coupled with animals migrating to eat new fruit; so when all of those aspects disappeared, so did the virus in whatever carrier it was in.

It is possible that a treetop species such as A. africanus could be important to the cycle. Historical information about the spread of Yellow Fever includes the actions of tree-cutters dropping tall trees and being attacked by treetop species of the mosquitoes being the exposure for their infection. Likewise, NHPs that dwell in the treetops have been infected with Yellow fever and then moved onto the ground in and around villages where additional species of mosquitoes fed on them allowing the virus to circulate in more species of mosquitoes. Incidentally, yellow fever is known to be active during rainy seasons, but with increase in disease incidence at the start of the dry season just like Ebola (Harper, 2004).

Some observations suggest that arthropods could transmit Ebola to humans. One study done in 1968 showed that Marburg, a related filovirus, could remain persistent in Aedes species for 3 weeks after experimental inoculation. That is not to say the virus replicated in the mosquito, or its salivary glands which is what occurs and is important in other mosquito-borne illnesses. Turrell and colleagues studied virus replication in arthropods in 1996 where they concluded that no virus replicated in the insects, but they also did not use the outbreak strains of Ebola to do the study, they used

Reston Ebola (Waterman, 1999; Turrell, Bressler & Rossi, 1996).

Still in the tree tops, Western Colobus Monkeys have been the focus of many Ebola infections among NHPs. This species lives in the canopies of trees and are strictly vegetarians (Kuhn & Calisher, 2008). It is probable that they are exposed to urine and/or feces of reservoir bats, or that they eat unfinished fruit left by bats sharing the canopy with them. If mosquitoes are involved somehow, that could be additive to the focus with these NHPs.

The dry season in Ebola-endemic areas of Africa runs from November to February, generally. This season coincides with large amounts of fruit ripening. Before the fruit all ripen, it is logical to presume that the animals are eating some other foods and then as the fruits ripen, there is competition for those fruits (Atherstone, Roesel & grace, 2014). When bats eat their fruit, they mash it with their teeth and suck the juices from it. When they are finished with a fruit, they spit out that pulp and drop any remaining fruit, making it available for other animals to ingest. The relevance of their chewing on soft wood for moisture is not understood, but it is notable (African Wildlife Foundation, 2014; Wildscreen Archive, 2014; Atherstone, Roesel & grace, 2014).

Many animals share the environment with bats from ground level. It is plausible to note other animals that have been found with antibodies or antigen for Ebola could have eaten contaminated fruit spit out or dropped by bats as their means of exposure. Animals noted in the literature for Ebola positive test results either by their infection or antibodies include dogs, chimps, gorillas, duikers, antelope, certain rodents and guinea pigs as well as pigs. Guinea pigs are not susceptible to infection and disease with wild-type Ebola viruses and when they are used in research, the viruses have to be adapted to guinea pigs in order to observe the disease and its processes (Wong et al., 2015). Additionally, following epizootic outbreaks of Ebola, animals found dead (often in groups) were bush pigs, porcupines and civet cats (Allela et al., 2005; Kuhn & Calisher, 2008).

Transmission between pigs and a reservoir animal could take place due to shared environment where exposure to feces of bats or other yet to be identified reservoirs, sharing of food scraps contaminated by saliva containing Ebola, or other interactions. A scenario might be where a hunter killed a bat that was unexpectedly viremic and fed the unwanted organs to his pigs. Any meat harvested from those pigs that was simply smoked or dried would pose risks to anyone handling and eating it especially without additional cooking to at least 60°C for 30-60 minutes or boiling the meat in tiny pieces for five minutes or more, allowing the internal temperatures to deactivate the virus thoroughly (Kuhn & Calisher, 2008).

With pigs as a component to outbreaks of Ebola, any butchering or care of pigs deemed vulnerable due to environmental potential exposure to wild reservoirs could potentiate human exposures. Disposal of any slaughter waste would be infectious and should not be recycled to feed other animals as has been noted during the discovery of prion diseases like Mad-Cow Disease. As mentioned above, even rumors of potential porcine diseases will prompt farmers to sell their stock of pigs faster, making spread – if infected, more problematic. Makerere University studied the movement of sick pigs and those pigs in contact with sick pigs where transport in excess of 500km occurred. If those pigs had been sick with Ebola, this transport would have moved the disease to many other distant regions (Atherstone, Roesel & grace, 2014).

There are some species of indigenous pigs in Africa; Uganda has Hylochoerus meinerthageni (giant forest hogs), Potamochoerus porcus (Red River Hogs), Potamochoerus larvatus (bush pigs), and Potamochoerus africanus (common warthogs). Some of these species have been observed to have wide geographic distributions and have been observed to breed with domestic species of pigs (Atherstone, Roesel & grace, 2014). It is possible for these wild species of pigs to periodically share habitats with reservoir species carrying Ebola which would provide means of exposure to domestic pigs.

Use as a Biological Weapon

It is documented that the Japanese terror group, Aum Shinrikyo, attempted to biomine the Ebola virus from an African outbreak at one point but they were not successful in doing so (Borio et al., 2002). Biomining of a virus would require those individuals attempting to collect samples of the virus to either acquire a dead infected animal or to covertly work alongside of medical personnel in an Ebola clinic and preserve the samples for later use which would likely require the shipping of the samples to a predetermined location or lab. The details of how this would be done will not be covered here for reasons of protecting global security. Anyone interested in culturing Ebola virus for use as a weapon would need sophisticated and expensive equipment and lab environments as well as specialized knowledge in virology, culturing techniques, safety and more. It is doubtful that less than a state-sponsored lab could be successful (Leitenberg & Zilinskas, 2012; Borio et al., 2002).

The head of the Department of Infectious Diseases at the FMBA's Institution of Advanced Training, Vladimir Nikiforov, says it is entirely possible to use Ebola as a weapon and he goes on to say, "Actually, this virus can be used in the form of a spray, which can lead to very big trouble." Other experts are concerned with the use of Ebola in a dirty-bomb situation, but in order for that to be practical, the design would have to shield the virus samples from heat so the heat of the blast did not kill the virus before dispersal. State sponsored labs have worked with this, but it will not be covered here (TV-Novosti, 2014).

In September, 2014 an Air Marshal was in a Nigerian airport awaiting his flight to Texas when an unknown man attacked him with a syringe. News reports say that they doubt the attacker knew who this man was and that the attacker fled the scene, but this feeds fears of this sort of attack using Ebola in a syringe to infect others deliberately. Fortunately for him, the syringe used in this attach did not contain deadly pathogens (Costello, Dienst & Gittens, 2014; Lozano, 2014).

More recent concerns about groups like ISIS that would try suicide like missions using Ebola infection as their means for terrorism have surfaced. There are a variety of articles circulating that suggest ISIS has sent groups to endemic areas to deliberately become infected to this end. There are analysts and national security experts who agree and say there have been intelligence reports that revealed ISIS members researching biological warfare, although not specifically Ebola (Dorminey, 2014; Dvorin, 2014).

There was more research suggested on Marburg in Soviet Russia through their biological warfare program, Biopreparat (code named Ferment). There were many institutions involved in the weaponizing of various microbes through that program but the main one working on filoviruses was Vector Lab in Novosibirsk. Vector researchers were able to perfect drying and milling of Marburg viruses to the desirable 1-5 micron size that is considered to be successful as an airborne agent. Although they worked on engineering of Marburg, they were not successful in genetically engineering it because of the templating needed in the case of RNA viruses using DNA templates which was not available as it would now be through gene banking. Vector research on Venezuelan Equine Encephalitis provides something useful related to Ebola for vaccine research and that is; because an infection that enters the body via aerosols and the respiratory system requires the immune system to protect the olfactory nerve which allows access to the brain where even vaccinated induction of the immune system does not provide protection. Because of this information, it seems prudent to discover Ebola transmission possibilities over neural pathways (Leitenberg & Zilinskas, 2012). Additionally, the delivery of a drug that inhibits the replication of Ebola which could be administered as an aerosol in a similar way to how Ribavirin is used to treat children for Respiratory Syncytial virus could prove useful and effective.

If Ebola were to be successfully used as a biological weapon it might be difficult to determine that while the outbreak is ongoing in Africa because healthcare facilities and those on frontlines for care and identification of the disease are rigorously training for travel related and contact-related cases. It might prove to be elusive if the disease were dispersed as an aerosol or by other air-dispersed means that exposed a great number of people which would certainly prolong accurate diagnosis and containment, and likely result in greater numbers of exposed in the healthcare environments. Additionally, the suspicion of a biological weaponized viral hemorrhagic fever would not be sufficient for a diagnosis, there would need to be an identification of the specific agent to at least Genus for treatment to be fully effective. Even today, 38 years after the first outbreaks, laboratory testing that can be utilized to diagnose cases remains unfortunately slow. Testing devices that could prove useful in the current outbreak are somehow stalled in production rather than being put to test and use where they are needed most. More than forty years after the first outbreak, samples are still being sent out of Africa and at the least, many miles from the clinic of origin to be tested and confirmed as positive or negative and those tests often require a second and even third test to be confirmatory due to the nature of the tests and the specificity relating to the virus, RNA, antigen or antibody the test targets for its result. It is hopeful that with the influx of many military troops from the U.S., U.K., China, and other countries that the testing of samples might be made more expedient and results more timely (Borio et al; 2002).

###

Thank you for taking the time to read this book. If you feel that you benefitted from this please take a moment to leave a review for me at your favorite retailer's website.

Kindest regards,

Leah E. Roberts

Bibliography

1. AABB. (2014, September). *Infection control for handling blood specimens from suspected ebola patients*. Retrieved from http://www.aabb.org/press/Pages/Infection-Control-for-Handling-Blood-Specimens-from-Suspected-Ebola-Patients.aspx

2. African Wildlife Foundation. (2014). *Bat: Eidolon helvum*. Retrieved from http://www.awf.org/wildlife-conservation/bat

3. Agenda for Environment and Responsible Development. (2009, May). *Needs assessment for hospitals in African countries in relation to infectious waste treatment*. Retrieved from http://gefmedwaste.org/downloads/Report:%20Needs%20Assessment%20for%20Hospitals%20in%20African%20Countries%20in%20Relation%20to%20Infectious%20Waste%20Treatment.pdf

4. Allela, L. O. I. S., Bourry, O., Pouillot, R., Delicat, A., Yaba, P., Kumulungui et al. (2005, March). Ebola virus antibody prevalence in dogs and human risk. *Emerging Infectious Diseases, 113*(3), 385-390.

5. Amoran, O. E., & Onwube, O. O. (2013, December 1). Infection control and practice of standard precautions among healthcare workers in northern Nigeria. *Journal of Global Infectious Diseases, 5*(4), 156-163.

6. Anand, V., Duffy, B., Yang, Z., Dejneka, N. S., Maguire, A. M., & Bennett, J. (2001, December 6). A deviant immune response to viral proteins and transgene product is generated on subretinal administration of adenovirus and adeno-associated virus. *Molecular Therapy, 5*(125). Retrieved from http://www.nature.com/mt/journal/v5/n2/full/mt200220a.html

7. Anderson, A. (2014). *The African concept of death* [Encyclopedia of death and dying]. Retrieved from http://www.deathreference.com/A-Bi/African-Religions.html

8. Associated Newspapers LTD. (2014, July 29). *In boiling hot suits with silent death lurking everywhere and the fear that a mistake could be fatal: Doctors give a gripping insight into their battle in the crucible of the biggest ebola outbreak in history.* Retrieved from http://www.dailymail.co.uk/news/article-2710174/In-stifling-hot-suits-silent-death-lurking-fear-mistake-fatal-Brave-doctors-terrifying-insight-battle-crucible-biggest-Ebola-outbreak-history.html

9. Atherstone, C., Roesel, K., & Grace, D. (2014). *Ebola risk assessment in the pig value chain in Uganda* (International Livestock Research Institute). Retrieved from https://cgspace.cgiar.org/bitstream/handle/10568/41667/rr34.pdf?sequence=1

10. Baggi, F. M., Taybi, A., Kurth, A., Van Herp, M., Di Caro, A., Wölfel, R. et al. (2014, December 11). Management of pregnant women infected with ebola

virus in a treatment centre in Guinea, June 2014. *Eurosurveillance, 19*(49). Retrieved from http://www.eurosurveillance.org/ViewArticle.aspx?ArticleId=20983

11. Baize et al. (2014, April 16). Emergence of Zaire ebola virus disease in Guinea - preliminary report. *New England Journal of Medicine.* Retrieved from http://www.nejm.org/doi/full/10.1056/NEJMoa1404505#t=article

12. Barbeito, M. S., Mathews, C. T., & Taylor, L. A. (1967, March 6). Microbiological laboratory hazard of bearded men. *Applied Microbiology, 15*(4), 899-906. Retrieved from http://www.ncbi.nlm.nih.gov/pmc/articles/PMC547091/pdf/applmicro00234-0219.pdf

13. Baschiera, D. (2014, November 25). *Ebola outbreak: Darwin volunteer writes from Sierra Leone treatment centre, 'I just cry in my goggles'* [Convalescing patient re-infected after returning home]. Retrieved from http://www.abc.net.au/news/2014-11-26/darwin-ebola-volunteer-dan-baschiera-writes-from-sierra-leone/5919516

14. Baum, S. (2014, September 15). *Nebraska medical center uses telemedicine to treat ebola virus patient*. Retrieved from http://medcitynews.com/2014/09/nebraska-medical-center-uses-telemedicine-treat-ebola-virus-patient/

15. Baxter, A. (2000, June 24). Symptomless infection with ebola. *The Lancet, 355*(9222), 2178-2179. Retrieved from

http://www.sciencedirect.com/science/article/pii/S0140673600023941
16. Belluz, J. (2014, October 13). *A top scientist worries that Ebola has mutated to become more contagious*. Retrieved from http://www.vox.com/2014/10/13/6959087/ebola-outbreak-virus-mutated-airborne
17. Bhadelia, N. (2014, October 26). *A Doctor's Diary: Encountering Chaos And Kindness In An Ebola Ward*. Retrieved from http://www.ideastream.org/news/npr/355119076
18. Biek, R., Walsh, P. D., Leroy, E. M., & Real, L. A. (2006, October 27). Recent common ancestry of Ebola Zaire virus found in bat reservoir. *PLoS Pathogens, 2*(10). Retrieved from http://www.ncbi.nlm.nih.gov/pmc/articles/PMC1626099/
19. Blake, M. (2014, August 29). *Dogs eating corpses of Ebola victims in Liberia. and now the deadly virus has reached Senegal*. Retrieved from http://www.dailymail.co.uk/news/article-2737684/Dogs-EATING-corpses-Ebola-victims-Liberia-health-teams-pile-bodies-shallow-grave-middle-night-locals-refused-permission-use-land.html
20. Bogoch, S., & Bogoch, E. S. (2011, August 22). Prediction of specific virus outbreaks made from the increased concentration of a new class of virus genomic peptides, replikins. *Nature Precedings.* Retrieved from http://precedings.nature.com/documents/6279/version/1/files/npre20116279-1.pdf

21. Borchert, M., Mutyaba, I., Van Kerhove, M. D., Lutwama, J., Luwaga, H., Bisoborwa, G. et al. (2011). Ebola haemorrhagic fever outbreak in Masindi District, Uganda: Outbreak description and lessons learned. *BMC Infectious Diseases, 11*(357). Retrieved from http://www.biomedcentral.com/1471-2334/11/357

22. Borio, L., Inglesby, T., Schmaljohn, A. L., Hughes, J. M., Jahrling Peter B., Ksiazek, T. et al. (2002, May 8). Hemorrhagic fever viruses as biological weapons medical and public health management. *American Medical Association, 287*(18), 2391-2405.

23. Borsanyi, A. (2014, October 8). *Marked increase in ebola gene replikin count in 2012 & 2013 predicted current ebola outbreak; does recent sharp drop in replikin count signal early end for the current ebola outbreak?* Retrieved from http://www.prnewswire.com/news-releases/marked-increase-in-ebola-gene-replikin-count-in-2012--2013-predicted-current-ebola-outbreak-does-recent-sharp-drop-in-replikin-count-signal-early-end-for-the-current-ebola-outbreak-278578691.html

24. Boseley, S. (2014, October 1). *First Ebola patient diagnosed in US won't be treated with ZMapp.* Retrieved from http://www.theguardian.com/world/2014/oct/01/first-ebola-patient-us-no-zmapp

25. Briese, T., Calisher, C., & Higgs, S. (2013, August 30). Viruses of the family bunyaviridae: Are all available isolates reassortants? *Virology, 446*(1-2), 207-216.

26. Brosseau, L. M., & Jones, R. (2014, September 17). *Commentary: Health workers need optimal respiratory protection for Ebola*. Retrieved from http://www.cidrap.umn.edu/news-perspective/2014/09/commentary-health-workers-need-optimal-respiratory-protection-ebola
27. Buhler, S., Roddy, P., Nolte, E., & Borchert, M. (2014, February). Clinical documentation and data transfer from ebola and marburg virus disease wards in outbreak settings: Health care workers' experiences and preferences. *Viruses, 6,* 927-937.
28. Caillot, J.-L., & Voiglio, E. (2008). First clinicalstudy of a new virus-inhibiting surgical glove. *Swiss Medical Weekly, 2008*(138), 18-22.
29. Callimachi, R. (2014, September 18). *Fear of Ebola drives mob to kill officials in Guinea*. Retrieved from http://www.nytimes.com/2014/09/19/world/africa/fear-of-ebola-drives-mob-to-kill-officials-in-guinea.html?_r=2
30. Canada: Immigration and Refugee Board of Canada. (2012, November 6). *Nigeria: Ritual whereby a widow drinks the water used to clean her husband's corpse; consequences for a widow's refusal to drink the water; whether a widow's refusal is interpreted by others as responsibility for her husband's death*. Retrieved from http://www.refworld.org/docid/50b4aa8c2.html
31. Cann, A. J. (2005). *Principles of molecular virology.* United Kingdom: Elsevier Inc.

32. CDC. (2014, August 5). *Diagnosis* [Ebola virus disease]. Retrieved from http://www.cdc.gov/vhf/ebola/diagnosis/
33. CDC. (2014, August 14). *Interim guidance for environmental infection control in hospitals for ebola virus*. Retrieved from http://www.cdc.gov/vhf/ebola/hcp/environmental-infection-control-in-hospitals.html
34. CDC. (2014, September 18). *Outbreaks chronology: Ebola hemorrhagic fever*. Retrieved from http://www.cdc.gov/vhf/ebola/resources/outbreak-table.html
35. Chang, F. K., Chen, M. L., Cheng, S. F., Shih, T. S., & Mao, I. F. (2007, May 23). Field protection effectiveness of chemical protective suits and gloves evaluated by biomonitoring. *Occup. Environ. Med., 2007*(64), 759-762.
36. Chen, C., & Kitamura, M. (2014, August 19). *Ebola orphans targeted by aid groups as newest victims.* Retrieved from http://www.bloomberg.com/news/2014-08-19/ebola-orphans-targeted-by-aid-groups-as-newest-victims.html
37. Chen, S. (2014, August 14). *Shenzen company develops kit to test for ebola virus, report says.* Retrieved from http://www.scmp.com/news/china/article/1573511/shenzhen-company-develops-kit-test-ebola-virus-report-says
38. Choi, J. H., Jonsson-Schmunk, K., Qui, X., Shedlock, D. J., Strong, J., Xu, J. X. et al. (2014,

November 1). A single dose respiratory recombinant adenovirus-based vaccine provides long-Term protection for non-Human primates from lethal ebola infection. *Mol. Pharmaceutics.* Retrieved from http://pubs.acs.org/doi/pdf/10.1021/mp500646d

39. Close, W. T. (2002). *Ebola: Through the eyes of the people.* USA: Meadowlark Springs Productions.

40. Coates, M. J., Jundi, A. S., & James, M. R. (2000). Chemical protective clothing; a study into the ability of staff to perform lifesaving procedures. *J. Accid. Emerg. Med., 2000*(17), 115-118.

41. Cohen, E. (2014, September 27). *Doctor treats Ebola with HIV drug in Liberia -- seemingly successfully.* Retrieved from http://www.cnn.com/2014/09/27/health/ebola-hiv-drug/

42. Cohen, E., Almasy, S., & Yan, H. (2014, October 13). *Texas nurse who had worn protective gear tests positive for Ebola.* Retrieved from http://www.cnn.com/2014/10/12/health/ebola/index.html

43. Coico, R., & Sunshine, G. (2009). *Immunology: A short course.* New Jersey: John Wiley & Sons, Inc.

44. Collingwood, J. (2007). *Tackling the fears of the 'worried well'* [Psych central]. Retrieved from http://psychcentral.com/lib/tackling-the-fears-of-the-worried-well/0001227

45. Costello, T., Dienst, J., & Gittens, H. (2014, September 8). *Air marshall attacked with syringe in Nigeria, flies to Texas.* Retrieved from

http://www.nbcnews.com/news/us-news/air-marshal-attacked-syringe-nigeria-flies-texas-n198691
46. Croteau, S. J. (2014, September 7). *Wife says Ebola-infected MD 'very sick' but improving*. Retrieved from http://www.telegram.com/article/20140907/NEWS/309079884/1116
47. Dimmit, D. (2014, June 9). *Hypochlorous acid for definitive terminal cleaning of the hospital environment*. Retrieved from http://www.infectioncontroltoday.com
48. Dorminey, B. (2014, October 5). *Ebola as ISIS bio-weapon?* Retrieved from http://www.forbes.com/sites/brucedorminey/2014/10/05/ebola-as-isis-bio-weapon/
49. Drew, J. (2012, November 20). *Method for preserving viral particles*. Retrieved from http://www.freepatentsonline.com/8313897.html
50. Drug Discovery and Development Magazine. (2014, July 31). *Replikin count predicts Ebola outbreaks*. Retrieved from http://www.dddmag.com/news/2014/07/replikin-count-predicts-ebola-outbreaks
51. Dudas, G., & Rambaut, A. (2014, May 2). Phylogenetic analysis of Guinea 2014 EBOV Ebolavirus outbreak. *PLoS Current Outbreaks.* Retrieved from http://currents.plos.org/outbreaks/article/phylogenetic-analysis-of-guinea-2014-ebov-ebolavirus-outbreak-2/
52. Dvorin, T. (2014, October 10). *Could ISIS target the West with Ebola?* Retrieved from

http://www.israelnationalnews.com/News/News.aspx/186020#.VDvayfldWSo
53. Ebola Deeply. (2015). *In Sierra Leone, sexual transmission of Ebola threatens to undermine progress*. Retrieved from
http://www.eboladeeply.org/articles/2015/01/7153/sierra-leone-sexual-transmission-ebola-threatens-undermine-progress/
54. Efstathiou, G., Papastavrou, E., Raftopoulos, V., & Merkouris, A. (2011). Factors influencing nurses' compliance with standard precautions in order to avoid occupational exposure to microorganisms: A focus group study. *BMC Nursing, 10*(1), 1-12. Retrieved from http://www.biomedcentral.com/1472-6955/10/1
55. Efstathiou, G., Papastavrou, E., Raftopoulos, V., & Merkouris, A. (2013, December 1). Prevalence of occupational exposure to pathogens and reporting behaviour among Cypriot nurses. *International Journal of Caring Sciences, 6*(3), 420-430.
56. Eveillard, M. (2011). Wearing gloves: The worst enemy of hand hygiene. *Future Microbiol., 6*(8), 835-837.
57. Fallah, S. (2014, December 9). *Fake death certificates spark Ebola's spread in Liberia*. Retrieved from
http://www.eboladeeply.org/articles/2014/12/6856/fake-death-certificates-spark-ebolas-spread-liberia/
58. Federation of American Scientists. (1998). *Section 3-biological weapons technology*. Retrieved from http://fas.org/irp/threat/mctl98-2/p2sec03.pdf

59. Flohr, L. (2013, January). *Ebola virus successfully transmitted from pigs to monkeys*. Retrieved from http://science-fare.com/article/ebola-virus-successfully-transmitted-pigs-monkeys

60. Fox News. (2014, September 19). *At least 8 Ebola aid workers reportedly killed 'in cold blood' by villagers in Guinea*. Retrieved from http://www.foxnews.com/world/2014/09/19/at-least-8-ebola-aid-workers-reportedly-killed-in-cold-blood-by-villagers-in/

61. Fox News. (2014, August 19). *South Carolina physician to combat Ebola in Liberia with disinfecting robots*. Retrieved from http://www.foxnews.com/health/2014/08/19/south-carolina-physician-taking-disinfecting-robots-to-liberia-to-combat-ebola/

62. Fox, M. (2015, January 19). *Genetically modified cattle with human DNA might hold ebola cure*. Retrieved from http://www.nbcnews.com/storyline/ebola-virus-outbreak/genetically-modified-cattle-human-dna-might-hold-ebola-cure-n287796

63. Francia, J. R. (2010). *A study of the Ebola virus glycoprotein: Disruption of host surface protein*, Cell & Molecular Biology, University of Pennsylvania. Retrieved from http://repository.upenn.edu/cgi/viewcontent.cgi?article=1295&context=edissertations

64. Gbadamosi, S., & Olukoya, O. (2014, August 31). *Ebola becoming harder to treat —US experts •It is taking toll on Nigeria's economy —OBJ*. Retrieved from

http://www.tribune.com.ng/news/top-stories/item/14787-ebola-becoming-harder-to-treat-us-experts-it-is-taking-toll-on-nigeria-s-economy-obj
65. Gettleman, J. (2014, December 13). *An Ebola orphan's plea in Africa: 'Do you want me?'* Retrieved from http://www.nytimes.com/2014/12/14/world/africa/an-ebola-orphans-plea-in-africa-do-you-want-me.html?_r=2
66. Ghana Web. (2014, September 22). *Cholera kills 12 in Cape Coast*. Retrieved from http://www.ghanaweb.com/GhanaHomePage/regional/artikel.php?ID=326921
67. Gignon, M., Farcy, S., Schmit, J. L., & Ganry, O. (2012). Prevention of healthcare-associated infections in general practice: Current practice and drivers for change in a French study. *Indian Journal of Medical Microbiology, 30*(1), 69-75.
68. Gire, S. K., Stremlau, M., Andersen, K. G., Schaffner, S. F., Bjornosn, Z., Rubins, K. et al. (2012, November 9). Emerging disease or diagnosis? *Science, 338*(6108), 750-752. Retrieved from http://www.sciencemag.org/content/338/6108/750.full
69. Global Medics. (2014). *Clinell universal wipes*. Retrieved from http://globalmedics.co.nz/media//Clinell_Universal_Wipes_Brochure_Low_Res.pdf
70. Grady, D. (2014, December 8). *An Ebola doctor's return from the edge of death*. Retrieved from http://timesofindia.indiatimes.com/world/us/An-Ebola-

doctors-return-from-the-edge-of-death/articleshow/45410146.cms
71. Grady, D., & Fink, S. (2014, August 9). *Tracing ebola's outbreak to an African 2-year-old*. Retrieved from http://www.nytimes.com/2014/08/10/world/africa/tracing-ebolas-breakout-to-an-african-2-year-old.html?_r=0
72. Graf, H. (2014, October 9). *Seattle scientist: Government 'underestimated' ebola*. Retrieved from http://www.king5.com/story/news/health/2014/10/09/seattle-scientist-says-us-government-underestimated-ebola/16956505/
73. Haglage, A. (2014, August 13). *Kissing the corpses in ebola country*. Retrieved from http://www.thedailybeast.com/articles/2014/08/13/kissing-the-corpses-in-ebola-country.html
74. Hainer, R. (2014). *The length of the gestation period in swine*. Retrieved from http://animals.pawnation.com/length-gestation-period-swine-3417.html
75. Han, G.-Z., & Worobey, M. (2011, August 4). Homologous recombination in negative sense RNA viruses. *Viruses, 357,* 1358-1373. doi:10.3390/v3081358
76. Harmon, W. Q. (2014, December 30). *Cremation abolished*. Retrieved from http://liberianobserver.com/news-development/cremation-abolished
77. Harper, T. K. (2004). *TKH virology notes: Yellow fever*. Retrieved from http://www.tarakharper.com/v_yellow.htm

78. Harriman, K. H., & Brosseau, L. (2011, April 28). *Controversy: Respiratory protection for healthcare workers*. Retrieved from http://www.medscape.com/viewarticle/741245_3
79. Hayden, E. C. (2014, September 24). *Infectious disease: Ebola's lost ward*. Retrieved from http://www.nature.com/news/infectious-disease-ebola-s-lost-ward-1.15990?WT.mc_id=TWT_NatureNews
80. Healio. (2014, October 19). *Ebola patient in Germany treated with novel bio-filtration device*. Retrieved from http://www.healio.com/infectious-disease/practice-management/news/online/%7B790adcc2-e953-4d9b-9391-c56d77a23342%7D/ebola-patient-in-germany-treated-with-novel-bio-filtration-device
81. Helio Infectious Disease News. (2014, November 7). *Novel bio-filtration device produced positive results in Ebola patient*. Retrieved from http://www.healio.com/infectious-disease/emerging-diseases/news/online/%7B5cc0b6f3-4008-4cdc-b556-d039f1b5bb1a%7D/novel-bio-filtration-device-produced-positive-results-in-ebola-patient
82. Hewlett, B., & Hewlett, B. (2008). *Ebola, culture and politics: The anthropology of an emerging disease.* California, USA: Thompson Wadsworth.
83. Homeland Security News Wire. (2014, September 23). *Concerns about use of Ebola as a bioweapon exaggerated: Experts*. Retrieved from http://www.homelandsecuritynewswire.com/dr201409

23-concerns-about-use-of-ebola-as-a-bioweapon-exaggerated-experts
84. Homeland Security News Wire (2). (2014, October 20). *21-day quarantine for ebola may not be enough to prevent spread of virus: Study*. Retrieved from http://www.homelandsecuritynewswire.com/dr20141020-21day-quarantine-for-ebola-may-not-be-enough-to-prevent-spread-of-virus-study
85. Howard, C. R. (2005). *Viral hemorrhagic fevers*. San Diego, CA: Elsevier Inc.
86. Hubner, N.-O., Goerdt, A.-M., Stanislawski, N., Assadian, O., Heidecke, C.-D., Kramer, A. et al. (2010, July 26). Bacterial migration through punctured surgical gloves under real surgical conditions. *BMC Infectious Diseases, 10*(92), 1-6. Retrieved from http://www.biomedcentral.com/1471-2334/10/192
87. Infectious Diseases Society of America. (2011, May 13). *Pigs susceptible to virulent ebolavirus can transmit the virus to other animals*. Retrieved from http://www.sciencedaily.com/releases/2011/05/110513064355.htm
88. International Society for Infectious Diseases. (2014, September 1). *Ebola virus disease - West Africa* [Email notification service containing daily updates]. Retrieved from http://www.promedmail.org/
89. IRIN News. (2014, December 18). *Mystery over Ebola survivors' ailments*. Retrieved from http://www.irinnews.org/report/100952/mystery-over-ebola-survivors-ailments

90. IRIN News. (2014, September 22). *West africa gears up to contain Ebola spread*. Retrieved from http://www.irinnews.org/report/100645/west-africa-gears-up-to-contain-ebola-spread
91. Iris, F. (2014, November). *Ebola: A speculative concept that could prove a direct avenue for the detection of an incipient outbreak*. Retrieved from http://www.bmsystems.net/download/Ebola-a-speculative-concept-that-could-rovide-a-direct-avenue-for-the-detection-of-an-incipient-outbreak-bmsystems05112014.pdf
92. Jane, S. G., Rosanna, F. P., Martin, D. C., Paul, D., Joanne, E. E., Tim, W. et al. (2010, February 1). [Discussion about the effectiveness of cleaning agents on microbes including enveloped viruses] Effectiveness of common household cleaning agents in reducing the viability of human influenza a/H1N1. Retrieved from http://www.plosone.org/article/info%3Adoi%2F10.1371%2Fjournal.pone.0008987
93. Jayalakshmi, K. (2014, October 16). *Ebola: WHO cites cases with longer incubation period of 42 days*. Retrieved from http://www.ibtimes.co.uk/ebola-who-cites-cases-longer-incubation-period-42-days-1470326
94. Johansen, L. M., Brannan, J. M., Delos, S. E., Shoemaker, C. J., Stossel, A., Lear, C. et al. (2013). FDA-Approved selective estrogen receptor modulators inhibit ebola virus infection. *Sci. Transl. Med., 5*(190), 190ra79. Retrieved from http://stm.sciencemag.org/content/5/190/190ra79.abstract

95. Johnson, A. M. (2014, November 27). *Liberia: Ebola doctor alarmed over male survivors infecting partners.* Retrieved from http://allafrica.com/stories/201411271023.html

96. Jones, R. M., & Brosseau, L. M. (2014, November 18). *Commentary: Ebola virus transmission via contact and aerosol — a new paradigm.* Retrieved from http://www.cidrap.umn.edu/news-perspective/2014/11/commentary-ebola-virus-transmission-contact-and-aerosol-new-paradigm

97. Journeyman Pictures. (2014, August 26). *Fighting to contain Sierra Leone's ebola epidemic* [Video]. Retrieved from https://www.youtube.com/watch?v=jTF7i6OBGQk&feature=youtu.be

98. Kempner, M. (2014, November 7). *As more survive Ebola, questions about sexual transmission arise.* Retrieved from http://rhrealitycheck.org/article/2014/11/07/survive-ebola-questions-sexual-transmission-arise/

99. Kennedy, J., Bek, J., & Griffin, D. (2000, September). Selection and use of disinfectants. *NebGuide.* Retrieved from http://extension.unl.edu/publications

100. King, J. W., Khan, A. A., Cunha, B. A., Kerkering, T. M., Malik, R., & Talavera, F. (2014, September 4). *Ebola virus infection treatment & management.* Retrieved from http://emedicine.medscape.com/article/216288-treatment

101. Kobinger, G. P., Leung, A., Neufeld, J., Richardson, J. S., Falzarano, D., Smith, G. et al. (2011, May 12). Replication, pathogenicity, shedding, and transmission of Zaire ebolavirus in pigs. *The Journal of Infectious Diseases, 204*(2), 200-208. Retrieved from http://jid.oxfordjournals.org/content/204/2/200

102. Korinth, G., Schmid, K., Midasch, O., Boettcher, M. I., Angerer, J., & Drexler, H. (2007, October). Investigations on permeation of mitomycin C through double layers of natural rubber gloves. *Ann. Occup. Hyg., 51*(7), 593-600.

103. Kreuels, B., Wichmann, D., Emmerich, P., Schmidt-Chanasit, J., de Heer, G., Kluge, S. et al. (2014, October 22). A case of severe ebola virus infection complicated by gram-negative septicemia. *The New England Journal of Medicine.*

104. Kuhn, J. H., & Calisher, C. H. (2008). *Filoviruses a compendium of 40 years of epidemiological, clinical, and laboratory studies.* Austria: Springer-Verlag/ Wein.

105. Lagow, B. (2002). *PDR guide to biological and chemical warfare response.* Montvale, NJ: Thompson PDR.

106. Leiss, J. K., Sousa, S., & Boal, W. L. (2009, November 5). Circumstances surrounding occupational blood exposure events in the national study to prevent blood exposure in paramedics. *Industrial Health, 2009*(47), 139-144. Retrieved from http://www.ncbi.nlm.nih.gov/pubmed/19367042

107. Leitenberg, M., & Zilinskas, R. (2012). *The Soviet biological weapons program a history.* Cambridge, Mass: Harvard University Press.
108. Leroy, E. M., Telfer, P., Kumulungui, B., Yaba, P., Rouquet, P., Roques, P. et al. (2004, December 1). A serological survey of ebola virus infection in central African nonhuman primates. *Journal of Infectious Diseases, 190,* 1895-1899. Retrieved from http://www.jhsph.edu/research/affiliated-programs/walter-reed-johns-hopkins-cameroon-program/documents/Papers/EbolaSerology.pdf
109. Leroy, E., Baize, S., Volchkov, V., Fisher-Hoch, S., Georges-Courbot, M., Lansoud-Soukate, J. et al. (2000, June 24). Human asymptomatic Ebola infection and strong inflammatory response. *Lancet, 355*(9222), 2210-5. Retrieved from http://www.ncbi.nlm.nih.gov/pubmed/10881895
110. Leroy, E. M., Baize, S., Mavoungou, E., & Apetrei, C. (2002, August). Sequence analysis of the GP, NP, VP40 and VP24 genes of. *Journal of General Virology, 2002*(83), 67-73. Retrieved from http://www.eva.mpg.de/primat/ebola_workshop/pdf/Leroy_et_alGabon96phylogeny.pdf
111. Leroy, E. M., Epelboin, A., Mondonge, V., Pourrut, X., Gonzalez, J.-P., Muyembe-Tamfum, J.-J. et al. (2009). Human Ebola outbreak resulting from the direct exposure to fruit bats in Luebo, Democratic Republic of Congo, 2007. *Vector-Borne and Zoonotic Diseases, 9*(6200), 723-731. Retrieved from

http://online.liebertpub.com/doi/pdfplus/10.1089/vbz.2008.0167
112. LiverTox. (2014, September 10). *Drug record lamivudine*. Retrieved from http://livertox.nih.gov/Lamivudine.htm
113. Lozano, J. A. (2014, September 9). *FBI says syringe used to attack US air marshal in Nigeria did not contain deadly pathogens*. Retrieved from http://health.usnews.com/health-news/news/articles/2014/09/09/fbi-air-marshal-attacked-with-syringe-in-nigeria
114. Lupi, O., & Tyring, S. K. (2003, December 1). Tropical dermatology: Viral tropical diseases. *Journal of the American Academy of Dermatology,* pp. 979-1002. doi:10.1016/S0190-9622(03)02728-2
115. Lupkin, S. (2014, August 29). *Ebola outbreak spreads: Senegal reports 1st case*. Retrieved from http://abcnews.go.com/Health/senegal-reports-1st-ebola-case-outbreak-continues/story?id=25177554
116. Lydersen, K. (2014, December 9). *Ebola teams need better cultural understanding, anthropologists say.* Retrieved from http://blogs.discovermagazine.com/crux/2014/12/09/ebola-cultural-anthropologists/#.VJMRVV4AKB
117. Mark, M. (2014, September 8). *Ebola orphans in Sierra Leone face isolation from hard-hit relatives.* Retrieved from http://www.theguardian.com/global-development/2014/sep/08/ebola-orphans-sierra-leone-isolation-families

118. Mark, M. (2014, September 20). *'Ebola makes you a risk to yourself: Touching your face can infect you.'* Retrieved from http://www.theguardian.com/world/2014/sep/21/ebola-makes-you-a-risk-to-yourself-sierra-leone
119. McCordic, C. (2014, August 26). *Ebola frontline: Life inside a quarantined village*. Retrieved from http://www.newsweek.com/ebola-frontline-inside-quarantined-village-locals-suffer-266849
120. Medecins Sans Frontieres. (2014, September 5). *Ebola: Eric's last walk*. Retrieved from http://www.msf.org/article/ebola-erics-last-walk
121. Medecins Sans Frontieres. (2014, September 16). *Liberia: The boy who tricked ebola*. Retrieved from http://www.msf.org/article/liberia-boy-who-tricked-ebola
122. Millar, K. (2014, August 26). *Ebola's victims: Not just those it infects*. Retrieved from http://www.mhtf.org/2014/08/26/ebolas-victims-not-just-those-it-infects/
123. Mis, M. (2014, September 5). *West africa: Could there be a positive note to the ebola outbreak?* Retrieved from http://allafrica.com/stories/201409051608.html
124. Mobula, L. M. (2014, October 13). Courage is not the absence of fear: Responding to the ebola outbreak in Liberia. *Global Health Science and Practice,* pp. 1-3.
125. Netburn, D. (2014, August 28). *The most complete ebola genome yet: What it can tell us.*

Retrieved from http://www.latimes.com/science/la-sci-ebola-genome-20140829-story.html#page=1
126. Neuman, S. (2014, October 8). *Dallas Ebola patient Thomas Eric Duncan has died.* Retrieved from http://www.npr.org/blogs/thetwo-way/2014/10/08/354577799/dallas-ebola-patient-thomas-eric-duncan-dies-hospital-says
127. New Atlantis Full Documentaries. (2013, May 30). *Ebola: The world's most dangerous virus (full documentary).* Retrieved from https://www.youtube.com/watch?v=w-bC6pfzxxo
128. Nossiter, A. (2014, September 22). *Fresh graves point to undercount of Ebola toll.* Retrieved from http://www.nytimes.com/2014/09/23/world/africa/23ebola.html?_r=1
129. Olival, K. J., & Hayman, D. T. S. (2014, April 17). Filoviruses in bats: Current knowledge and future directions. *Viruese, 6*(4), 1759-1788.
130. Onishi, N. (2014, October 1). *U.S. patient aided pregnant Liberian, then took ill.* Retrieved from http://www.nytimes.com/2014/10/02/world/africa/ebola-victim-texas-thomas-eric-duncan.html?_r=0
131. OSHA. (2014, October). *Standards* [Occupational safety standards]. Retrieved from https://www.osha.gov/SLTC/ebola/standards.html
132. Pattyn, S. R. (1978). *Ebola hemorrhagic fever.* Amsterdam, The Netherlands: Slsevier/North-Holland.
133. PBS. (2014, September 9). *Ebola outbreak* [Frontline documentary]. Retrieved from

http://www.pbs.org/wgbh/pages/frontline/ebola-outbreak/
134. Piercy, T. J., Smither, S. J., Steward, J. A., Eastaugh, L., & Lever, M. S. (2010, May 22). The survival of filoviruses in liquids, on solid substrates and in a dynamic aerosol. *Journal of Applied Microbiology, 109*(5), 1531-1539. Retrieved from http://onlinelibrary.wiley.com/doi/10.1111/j.1365-2672.2010.04778.x/full
135. Pigott, D. M., Golding, N., Mylne, A., Huang, Z., Henry, A. J., Weiss, D. J. et al. (2014, September 8). Mapping the zoonotic niche of Ebola virus disease in Africa. *ELife, 3*(e04395), 1-29.
136. Pinzon, J. E., Wilson, J. M., Tucker, C. J., Arthur, R., Jahrling, P. B., & Formenty, P. (2004, November). Trigger events: Enviroclimatic coupling of Ebola hemorrhagic fever outbreaks. *American Journal of Tropical Medicine and Hygiene, 71*(5), 664-674. Retrieved from http://www.ajtmh.org/content/71/5/664.long
137. Pourrut, X., Kumulungui, B., Wittman, T., Moussavou, G., Delicat, A., Yaba, P. et al. (2005, June). The natural history of ebola virus in Africa. *Microbes and Infection, 7*(7-8), 1005-1014. Retrieved from http://www.sciencedirect.com/science/article/pii/S1286457905001437
138. Prince, H., & Prince, D. L. (2001). *Disinfection, sterilization, and preservation fifth edition.* USA: Lippincott Williams & Wilkins.

139. PRNewswire. (2014, December 29). *Roche receives FDA emergency use authorization for the LightMix® Ebola Zaire rRT-PCR test.* Retrieved from http://www.prnewswire.com/news-releases/roche-receives-fda-emergency-use-authorization-for-the-lightmix-ebola-zaire-rrt-pcr-test-300014109.html
140. Public Health Agency of Canada. (2014). *Ebolavirus pathogen safety data sheet-infectious substances*. Retrieved from http://www.phac-aspc.gc.ca/lab-bio/res/psds-ftss/ebola-eng.php
141. Recombinomics. (2007, November 15). *Ebola recombination* [Commentary].
142. Reddy, S. (2014, December 15). *The 20% who spread most disease*. Retrieved from http://www.wsj.com/articles/the-20-who-spread-most-disease-1418686476
143. Reiter, P., Turell, M., Coleman, R., Miller, B., Maupin, G., Liz, J. et al. (1999). Field Investigations of an Outbreak of Ebola Hemorrhagic Fever, Kikwit, (Supplement 1, Vol. 179, pp. s148-s154). Retrieved from http://jid.oxfordjournals.org/content/179/Supplement_1/S148.full.pdf
144. Reuters. (2014, September 19). *Timeline - worst Ebola outbreak on record tests global response*. Retrieved from http://in.reuters.com/article/2014/09/19/health-ebola-idINKBN0HE04520140919
145. Rodriguez, L. L., Roo, A. D., Guimard, Y., Trappier, S. G., Sanchez, A. B., D., Williams, A. J. et al. (1999). Persistence and Genetic Stability of Ebola Virus

during the Outbreak in Kikwit, Democratic Republic of the Congo, 1995. *The Journal of Infectious Diseases, 179*(Supplement 1), S170-S176. Retrieved from http://jid.oxfordjournals.org/content/179/Supplement_1/S170.long

146. Romualdo dos Santos, T. C., Roseira, C. E., Batista Dias Passos, I. P., & Moralez de Figueiredo, R. (2013, November). The use of gloves by nursing staff: Transmission risk protection. *Journal of Nursing, 7*(11), 6438-45.

147. Ryabchikova, E. I., & Price, B. B. S. (2004). *Ebola and marburg viruses a view using electron microscopy.* Columbus, OH: Battelle Press.

148. Saez, A. M., & et al. (2014, December 10). Investigating the zoonotic origin of the West African Ebola epidemic. *EmBO Molecular Medicine.* Retrieved from http://onlinelibrary.wiley.com/doi/10.15252/emmm.201404792/pdf

149. Sanchez, A., & Rollin, P. (2005, October). Complete genome sequence of an Ebola virus (Sudan species). *Virus Research, 113*(1), 16-25.

150. Sanchez, A., Wagoner, K. E., & Rollin, P. (2007). Sequence-Based human leukocyte antigen—B typing of patients infected with ebola virus in Uganda in 2000: Identification of alleles associated with fatal and nonfatal disease outcomes. *The Journal of Infectious Diseases, 196*(2), S329-S336. Retrieved from http://jid.oxfordjournals.org/content/196/Supplement_2/S329.long

151. Sanchez, R. (2014, August 29). *Senegal confirms first Ebola case*. Retrieved from http://www.cnn.com/2014/08/29/health/ebola-outbreak-senegal/

152. Schieffelin, E. A. (2014, October 29). Clinical illness and outcomes in patients with Ebola in Sierra Leone. *The New England Journal of Medicine.* Retrieved from http://www.nejm.org/doi/full/10.1056/NEJMoa1411680#t=articleTop

153. schülke. (2014). *Kodan wipes*. Retrieved from http://www.schuelke.com/download/pdf/cint_lint_kodan_wipes_prod.pdf

154. ScienceDaily. (2011, May 13). *Pigs susceptible to virulent ebolavirus can transmit the virus to other animals*. Retrieved from http://www.sciencedaily.com/releases/2011/05/110513064355.htm

155. ScienceDaily. (2014, April 22). *Researchers identify a new variant of Ebola virus in Guinea*. Retrieved from http://www.sciencedaily.com/releases/2014/04/140422113349.htm

156. Sencan, I., Sahin, I., Yildirim, M., & Yesildal, N. (2004, February). Unrecognized abrasions and occupational exposures to blood-borne pathogens among health care workers in Turkey. *Occupational Medicine, 2004*(54), 202-206.

157. Shirai, J., Kanno, T., Tsuchiya, Y., Mitsubayashi, S., & Seki, R. (2000, January). Effects of chlorine, iodine,

quaternary ammonium compound disinfectants on several exotic disease viruses. *J. Vet. Med. Sci., 62*(1), 85-92.
158. Simmonds, J. H. (2014). *Cleaning for health.* Retrieved from http://www.cleaning-for-health.org/disinfectant-chart/
159. Smallstarter ThinkTank. (2013, August 23). *Pig farming – how this business is changing lives in Africa and everything you need to start your own.* Retrieved from http://www.smallstarter.com/browse-ideas/agribusiness-and-food/how-to-start-pig-farming-in-africa
160. Smith-Spark, L., & Perez Maestro, L. (2014, October 8). *Spanish nurse's assistant may have caught Ebola taking off suit, doctor says.* Retrieved from http://www.cnn.com/2014/10/08/world/europe/ebola-spain/index.html
161. Snyder, R. E., & Marlow, M. A. (2014, October 30). Ebola in urban slums: The elephantin the room. *The Lancet.* Retrieved from http://download.thelancet.com/pdfs/journals/lancet/PIIS2214109X14703390.pdf
162. Sompayrac, L. (2008). *How the immune systen works 3rd edition.* Massachusetts, USA: Blackwell Publishing.
163. Steenhuysen, J. (2014, September 24). *Insight-US hospitals unprepared to handle Ebola waste.* Retrieved from http://in.reuters.com/article/2014/09/24/health-ebola-usa-hospitals-idINL2N0RP00E20140924

164. Stephen, K. G., Augustine, G., Kristian, G. A., Rachel, S. G. S., Daniel, J. P., Lansana, K. et al. (2014, September 12). Genomic surveillance elucidates ebola virus origin and transmission during the 2014 outbreak. *Science, 345,* 1369-1372.
165. Stern, J. E. (2014, October). *Hell in the hot zone* [Article to be published in Oct 2014 Vanity Fair magazine]. Retrieved from http://www.vanityfair.com/politics/2014/10/ebola-virus-epidemic-containment
166. Stone, F. P. (2007). *The "worried well" response to CBRN events: Analysis and solutions* [The counterproliferation papers future warfare series no. 40 USAF Counterproliferation Center]. Retrieved from http://fas.org/irp/threat/cbw/worried.pdf
167. Stramer, S. L. (2009, August). Ebola virus. *Transfusion, 49*(Supplement 1), 72S-74S. Retrieved from http://www.aabb.org/tm/eid/Documents/72s.pdf
168. Swaminathan, A., Martin, R., Gamon, S., Aboltins, C., Athan, E., Braitberg, G. et al. (2007, October). Personal protective equipment and antiviral drug use during hospitalization for suspected avian or pandemic influenza. *Emerging Infectious Diseases, 13*(10), 1541-1547.
169. Swanepoel, R., Leman, P. A., Burt, F. J., Zachariades, N. A., Braack, L. E., Ksiazek, T. G. et al. (1996, December 1). Experimental inoculation of plants and animals with ebola virus. *Emerging Infectious Diseases, 2*(4), 321-325. Retrieved from

http://www.ncbi.nlm.nih.gov/pmc/articles/PMC2639914/pdf/8969248.pdf
170. Tafilaku, J. (2013, November 20). *Immune privilege sites: Bringing down the barriers of regenerative medicine*. Retrieved from http://triplehelixblog.com/2013/11/immune-privilege-sites-bringing-down-the-barriers-of-regenerative-medicine/
171. Tamba, G. T. (2014, December 29). *Liberia: Ebola corpse arrested, 2000 persons quarantined*. Retrieved from http://allafrica.com/stories/201412292655.html
172. Tan, D.-X., Reiter, R. J., & Manchester, L. C. (2014, September 27). Ebola virus disease: Potential use of melatonin as a treatment. *Journal of Pineal Research.* doi: 10.1111/jpi.12186
173. Tenenbaum, D. J. (2014, August 28). *Ebola's end: History's lessons*. Retrieved from http://whyfiles.org/2014/ebolas-end-historys-lessons/
174. The Pig Site. (2006a, April 18). *Basic pig husbandry - the weaner*. Retrieved from http://www.thepigsite.com/articles/1616/basic-pig-husbandry-the-weaner
175. The PigSite. (2014, August 22). *Ebola risk in the pig value chain in Uganda*. Retrieved from http://www.thepigsite.com/articles/4834/ebola-risk-assessment-in-the-pig-value-chain-in-uganda
176. Thompson, B. L., Dwyer, D. M., Ussery, X. T., Denman, S., Vacek, P., & Schwartz, B. (1997, February). Handwashing and glove use in a long-term care facility. *Infection Control and Hospital Epidemiology, 18*(2), 97-

103. Retrieved from
http://www.jstor.org/discover/10.2307/30142397?uid=3739600&uid=2&uid=4&uid=3739256&sid=21105012807903
177. Trenchard, T. (2014, December 15). *Survivors cope with new Ebola after-effects*. Retrieved from http://www.aljazeera.com/news/africa/2014/12/survivors-cope-with-new-ebola-after-effects-2014121573521561384.html
178. Truscott, W., & Friedman, K. (2014, September 19). *Kimberly-Clark Ebola virus disease (EVD) precautions brief: September 19, 2014* (Kimberly-Clark, pp. 1-11).
179. Turrell, M. J., Bressler, D. S., & Rossi, C. A. (1996). Short report: Lack of virus replication in arthropods after intrathoracic inoculation of Ebola Reston virus. *The American Journal of Tropical Medicine and Hygiene, 55*(1), 89-90. Retrieved from http://europepmc.org/abstract/med/8702028
180. TV-Novosti. (2014, September 21). *Ebola can be turned into bioweapon, Russian & UK experts warn*. Retrieved from http://rt.com/news/178992-ebola-biological-weapon-terrorists/
181. TV-Novosti. (2014, September 21). *Ebola can be turned into bioweapon, Russian & UK experts warn*. Retrieved from http://rt.com/news/178992-ebola-biological-weapon-terrorists/
182. UC Berkeley Events. (2014, August 28). *The 2014 ebola outbreak: Update on an unprecedented public health event* [Lecture]. Retrieved from

https://www.youtube.com/watch?v=WCM3HWslbDE&feature=youtu.be
183. UNICEF. (2014, September). *Ebola virus disease: Personal protective equipment and other Ebola-related supply update*. Retrieved from http://reliefweb.int/sites/reliefweb.int/files/resources/UNICEF_Ebola_SuppliesInformationNote_1Sept2014.pdf
184. UTMB. (2013, November 27). *3.02 - Isolation of Patients with an Emerging Infectious disease (EID) or a possible EID*. Retrieved from http://www.utmb.edu/policies_and_procedures/Non-IHOP/Healthcare_Epidemiology/03.02%20-%20Isolation%20of%20Patients%20with%20an%20Emerging%20Infectious%20Disease%20(EID)%20or%20a%20Possible%20EID.pdf
185. VICE News. (2014, June 26). *Monkey meat and the ebola outbreak in Liberia*. Retrieved from https://www.youtube.com/watch?v=XasTcDsDfMg&feature=youtu.be
186. Vinik, D. (2014, October 6). *Is Ebola here to stay? "that's our biggest fear."* Retrieved from http://www.newrepublic.com/article/119711/nanomix-produces-diagnostic-device-test-ebola-just-minutes
187. Vogel, G. (2014, August 29). Genomes reveal start of ebola outbreak [Viral sequences demonstrate how the disease spread in sierra leone]. *Science, 345*(6200), 989-990.
188. Wasserman, E. (2014, October 23). *Frenchscientists roll out rapid diagnostic test for Ebola*.

Retrieved from
http://www.fiercediagnostics.com/story/french-scientists-roll-out-rapid-diagnostic-test-ebola/2014-10-23?utm_campaign=AddThis&utm_medium=AddThis&utm_source=mailto#.VErAzBpS7Ck.mailto

189. Waterman, T. (1999). *Are insects ebola's natural reservoir?* Retrieved from
https://web.stanford.edu/group/virus/filo/insects.html

190. Weiss, M. (2014, September 3). *Ebola survivors: Hospital staff exposed in Africa*. Retrieved from
http://bigstory.ap.org/article/missionary-infected-ebola-discuss-recovery

191. WHO. (2014, April). *Ebola virus disease* [Fact sheet]. Retrieved from
http://www.who.int/mediacentre/factsheets/fs103/en/

192. WHO. (2014). *Section 5 disinfect reusable supplies and equipment*. Retrieved from
http://www.who.int/csr/resources/publications/ebola/whoemcesr982sec5-6.pdf

193. Wildscreen Arkive. (2014). *Straw-colored fruit bat (Eidolon helvum)*. Retrieved from
http://www.arkive.org/straw-coloured-fruit-bat/eidolon-helvum/

194. Winnall, W., De Rose, R., Fernandez, C., Lloyd, S., Amarasena, T., Alcantara, S. et al. (2014). *Simian immunodeficiency virus (SIV) infection of the macaque testis - an immune privileged site*. Retrieved from
http://www.iasociety.org/Web/WebContent/File/HIV_Cure_Symposium_2014/Day_2/Abstracts/OA4-5.pdf

195. Wittman, T. J., Biek, R., Hassanin, A., Roquet, P., Reed, P., Yaba, P. et al. (2007, October 17). Isolates of Zaire ebolavirus from wild apes reveal genetic lineage and recombinants. *Microbiology, 104*(43), 17123-17127. Retrieved from http://www.ncbi.nlm.nih.gov/pmc/articles/PMC2040453/

196. Wolf, e. a. (2014, December 18). Severe Ebola virus disease with vascular leakage and multiorgan failure: Treatment of a patient in intensive care. *The Lancet.* Retrieved from http://www.thelancet.com/journals/lancet/article/PIIS0140-6736(14)62384-9/abstract#%2EVJqk-ekqfeQ%2Elinkedin

197. Wolz, A. (2014, September 18). Face to face with ebola-an emergency care center in Sierra Leone. *The New England Journal of Medicine, 371*(12), 1081-1083.

198. Wong, G., Qiu, X., Richardson, J., Cutts, T., Collington, B., Gren, J. et al. (2015, January). Ebola virus transmission in guinea pigs. *Journal of Virology, 89*(2), 1314-1323. Retrieved from http://jvi.asm.org/content/89/2/1314.full

199. World Health Organization. (2015, January 21). *Ebola situation report*. Retrieved from http://www.who.int/csr/disease/ebola/situation-reports/en/

200. Wynne, J. W., & Wang, L.-F. (2013, October 31). Bats and viruses: Friend or foe? *PLoS Pathogens, 9*(10). Retrieved from

http://www.plospathogens.org/article/info%3Adoi%2F10.1371%2Fjournal.ppat.1003651
201. Yang, S., Lee, G. W., Chen, C. M., Wu, C. C., & Yu, K. P. (2007, Winter). The size and concentration of droplets generated by coughing in human subjects. *Journal of Aerosol Medicine, 20*(4), 484-494. Retrieved from http://www.ncbi.nlm.nih.gov/pubmed/18158720
202. Yang, Z.-Y., Duckers, H., Sullivan, N. J., Sanchez, A., Nabel, E. G., & Nabel, G. J. (2000, June 27). Identification of the ebola virus glycoprotein as the main viral. *Nature America, Inc., 6*(8), 886-889. Retrieved from http://www.researchgate.net/publication/12388849_Identification_of_the_Ebola_virus_glycoprotein_as_the_main_viral_determinant_of_vascular_cell_cytotoxicity_and_injury/links/0912f50819afad7ec8000000
203. Youde, J. (2014, July 26). *The ebola outbreak in Guines, Liberia, and Sierra Leone*. Retrieved from http://www.e-ir.info/2014/07/26/the-ebola-outbreak-in-guinea-liberia-and-sierra-leone/
204. Young, Z. (2007, September 19). *Diary from DR Congo's Ebola frontline*. Retrieved from http://news.bbc.co.uk/2/hi/africa/7001506.stm
205. Zhang, G., & et al. (2012, December 20). Comparative analysis of bat genomes provides insight into the evolution of flight and immunity. *Science, 339*(6118), 456-460. Retrieved from http://www.sciencemag.org/content/339/6118/456.full
206. Zhin, Y. (2014, August 27). *Mass production of ebola test kits under way in China*. Retrieved from

http://www.chinatopix.com/articles/8093/20140827/mass-production-ebola-test-kits-underway-china.htm

www.ingramcontent.com/pod-product-compliance
Lightning Source LLC
Chambersburg PA
CBHW051807170526
45167CB00005B/1918
* 9 7 8 1 5 0 2 8 7 8 1 2 0 *